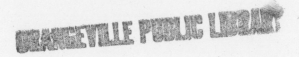

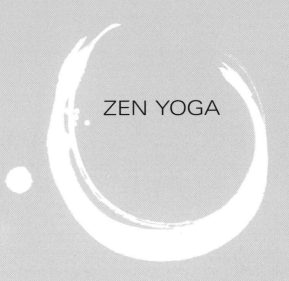

ZEN YOGA

ZEN YOGA

A Path to Enlightenment through Breathing,
Movement and Meditation

Aaron Hoopes

KODANSHA INTERNATIONAL
Tokyo • New York • London

Interior photography by KEVIN MURAKAMI
Additional interior shots by JESSE THOMPSON
Nature photography by YOJI OGURA
Calligraphy by KENHO UI

Distributed in the United States by Kodansha America, Inc., and in the United Kingdom and continental Europe by Kodansha Europe Ltd.

Published by Kodansha International Ltd., 17–14 Otowa 1-chome, Bunkyo-ku, Tokyo 112–8652, and Kodansha America, Inc.

Disclaimer: The author of this book does not dispense medical advice nor prescribe the use of any technique as a form of treatment for medical problems without the advice of a physician. The intent of the author is to offer information that is general in nature. The author and publisher assume no responsibility for your actions in the event you use the information in this book for yourself.

First edition, 2007
15 14 13 12 11 10 09 08 07   10 9 8 7 6 5 4 3 2 1

Library of Congress Cataloging-in-Publication Data

Hoopes, Aaron, 1963–
    Zen yoga : a path to Enlightenment through breathing, movement,
and meditation / Aaron Hoopes. — 1st ed.
        p. cm.
        ISBN-13: 978-4-7700-3047-4
1. Hatha yoga. 2. Zen Buddhism. I. Title.
RA781.7.H68 2007
613.7'046--dc22
                                2007012520

www.kodansha-intl.com

Close your eyes
and you will see clearly.

Cease to listen
and you will hear truth.

Be silent
and your heart will sing.

Seek no contacts
and you will find union.

Be still
and you will move forward.

Be gentle
and you will need no strength.

Be patient
and you will achieve all things.

Be humble
and you will remain whole.

—Sumnun

CONTENTS

PART 2   BODY

CHAPTER 3

Breathing Exercises   64

CHAPTER 4

Moving Exercises   84

PART 3 SPIRIT

INTRODUCTION
——What is Zen Yoga?

There are many paths
But the only one that leads
To the top of the mountain
Is the one you make yourself.

—Ancient Chinese saying

Zen Yoga: A Path to Enlightenment through Breathing, Movement, and Meditation is the culmination of more than twenty years of studying, training, and receiving instruction in various physical and spiritual arts of Japan, China, and India. It combines the mindful serenity of Zen meditation; the graceful, flowing movements of tai chi; the dynamic, energized breathing of qigong; and the peaceful stretching exercises of Shanti Yoga. Everyone has a body that can be moved in some manner, a mind that can be calmed to some extent, and a spirit that can be encouraged to develop. Zen Yoga is an art rather than a simple exercise program: it is a way to develop and refine oneself as a complete being.

Zen Yoga is a path to discovering the power that exists within you. It is a way of encouraging enlightenment and promoting harmony in your own life. It is a way of learning to radiate that harmony to all things you encounter. It is a way of living in full awareness of the present moment.

This book is intended to be much more than a series of pictures and explanations of yoga poses. Zen Yoga is a philosophy of life. The concepts are not new. Separately, most of the ideas put forward here have been around for thousands of years. They have been discussed and presented in much more eloquent words, by much more knowledgeable people than I. However, unless you have dedicated your life to one of the traditional martial arts of China or Japan, or have spent time in Nepal or Tibet, these philosophies can sometimes seem mysterious. They are often misunderstood. Within each true system of karate, kung fu, tai chi, yoga, or other Eastern art, there is a basic philosophy of living. I have spent my life working to integrate the disparate elements from those philosophies into a unified art that I call Zen Yoga.

I have written this book in the hope that some aspect of it will be of benefit to those on the journey of discovering themselves and how they fit into the larger picture. It is not a book only for martial artists seeking to advance their training. Nor is it a book solely for yoga adepts wanting new and different ways to stretch the body. At its most basic, it is a manual for anyone who desires to feel better and discover more about themselves.

Zen Yoga is a wonderfully simple process designed to make life more enjoyable through a coordinated integration of the body and mind. When the body and mind are connected, our spiritual nature is given the energy it needs to develop and flourish. This integrated state of being is accomplished through mindful awareness while practicing simple breathing, stretching, and relaxation exercises.

Practicing Zen Yoga is a noble endeavor. If you apply Zen Yoga to everything you do, you teach yourself to be successful in whatever you attempt. No matter whether you train in a different exercise system or discipline, or have not done any exercise for twenty years, I encourage you to apply the ideas found here to whatever you do. You will not be disappointed.

I wish you all the best on your journey in the hope that you realize your own perfection.

ZEN

First of all, what is Zen?

Well, Zen is…Zen is…Zen is….

Sorry, it's not that easy. As anyone who has looked into Zen knows, attempting to define Zen is like trying to catch a fish with your bare hands. It immediately slips between your fingers and wriggles away. The more you seek it, the harder it is to find. To say Zen is freedom, fluidity, or perfection is a start. Zen is right here, right now. Zen is this moment of existence. It is action without thought. It is thought and action as one. It is action before reaction.

Zen is Zen…though I know that's not helpful. Would saying that Zen is the reflection of the moon in a mountain stream leave you scratching your head?

The roots of Zen are found in ancient Chinese philosophy. The Chinese word for Zen is *ch'an*. In Sanskrit, the ancient language of India, it is *dhyana*, which can be roughly translated as pure human spirit. It can be imagined as the integration of the disparate aspects of the self into one complete and divine being. Zen was brought to Japan where Japanese Buddhists began to elaborate on it from the twelfth century. It eventually became the foundation of the code of Bushido, the way of the warrior. The samurai, who lived their lives at the edge of a sword and could die at any moment, were taught to concentrate on, and immerse themselves in, the here and now in order to connect with the fundamental core of their being. Doing so helped them develop their powers of concentration, self-control, awareness, and tranquility. If they approached each battle as if it were their last, they would be able to have every part of their being at their disposal.

Zen itself has no theory. It is not meditation. It is not thinking. It is not not-thinking. It is not something you learn. It is simply something you are. To practice Zen is to live fully and completely, not in the past or the future, but right here and right now. Zen *is*, in fact, the reflection of the moon in a mountain stream. It does not move, only the water flows by.

The use of Zen in this practice imparts a contemplative, mystical element to this process of self-discovery. The mindful awareness which Zen allows, and indeed encourages, offers a deeper exploration into your individual self.

YOGA

Yoga originated in India. The word is derived from the Sanskrit root *yug* meaning to join together and direct one's attention. It is the union of the body and mind with our spiritual nature. It is also the union of the individual with the universal spirit. It is both the goal and the path to realizing that goal.

At its most basic, yoga is any practice that allows practitioners to turn inward to find and experience their spiritual essence. By doing this they are able to impact more than just themselves. By bringing their own body, mind, and spirit into health and harmony, they can bring health and harmony to those around them and even to the world as a whole.

In the West, yoga is often considered to be a purely physical practice. But, in truth, it is much deeper than that. At times, in the study of yoga, the body has been likened to a temple. Yoga teaches the way to treat the body with reverence in order to give the spirit or soul a special place to reside and flourish. While this description is quite true, it is woefully inadequate. Yoga is a complete philosophy of living. It is mental as well as physical, psychological as well as spiritual. It teaches ethical discipline and the proper way of interacting within a society. It also teaches a way to turn inward and explore the inner core of one's being.

There are many different methods of practicing yoga. Some deal mainly with dynamic physical postures, while others concentrate primarily on breathing exercises. Still other yoga methods are devoted to chanting, reading, or worshiping. Finally, there are some that focus on deep meditation to help bring a sense of peace and serenity to daily life.

The underlying philosophy of yoga is that of wholeness: wholeness within the individual and wholeness in the individual's connection to the world. When there is coordination between the body, mind, and spirit, wholeness becomes holy. Not holy in a conventional religious sense but, rather, in terms of the connection to the divine part of us that exists within. The traditional yoga greeting *namaste* literally means "the divine within me greets the divine within you."

Very simply, yoga is about harnessing all the various aspects of individual existence and creating unity within.

On a grander scale, any spiritual practice or discipline that helps individuals awaken and realize their connection to something larger and more profound than their individual existence can be considered a yoga practice.

ZEN YOGA

Zen Yoga is a holistic system. It unites all aspects of the human self by meeting the fundamental needs of physical health, mental clarity, and spiritual peace. It is a spiritual discipline that is vast and profound.

It is Zen and it is yoga.

Zen Yoga is based on the peaceful stretching and breathing exercises of Shanti Yoga. Shanti Yoga was developed by Shanti Gowans, founder of the Shanti Yoga

Meditation Institute of Australia and author of more than fifteen books. It is non-stressful and encourages going at your own pace and only doing what is right for you. Everyone is different. We come in all shapes and sizes. Learning how your own body functions is of the utmost importance.

Zen Yoga is also based on the energized breathing and moving philosophy of Chinese qigong (pronounced *chē kung*) and tai chi. Qigong is the ancient Chinese practice of breathing exercises that fill the body with oxygen-rich blood and energy. Tai chi can be described as moving meditation. Its graceful, flowing movements encourage the circulation of energy.

Zen Yoga is also based on the mental serenity achieved through Zen meditation. Learning to calm the myriad thoughts that are continuously vying for attention within the mind allows us to think more clearly and with greater insight.

Zen Yoga also contains elements of various Eastern martial arts such as White Crane kung fu and Shotokan karate as well as some Western sports activities. Even if you are engaged in a different exercise system, Zen Yoga can be an invaluable supplement to your training.

But, most assuredly, Zen Yoga is much more than a set of physical exercises. Through the integration of body, mind, and spirit, Zen Yoga creates flexibility, health, vitality, and peace of mind.

The pace of modern life is characterized by hectic social and economic activity. We generate stress in our daily lives as our concentration is fractured and our energy is sapped. Exercise is put on the back burner because we are so caught up in all of the other things that are demanding our attention. Zen Yoga seeks to reverse this flow.

Its benefits include

- Stress relief

- Increased willpower

- Improved concentration

- Improved blood circulation and the release of toxins and impurities from the body

- Toning and strengthening of muscles

- Mindfulness

- More restful sleep

Even more important, by bringing into balance proper and effective breathing, movement, stretching, and deep relaxation practices, we can become aware of and learn to access the natural energy of the universe, called *chi* or *prana* (see next chapter).

Practicing Zen Yoga is not meant to be an aggressive or rigorous physical workout. Instead, it seeks to challenge you to realize your own potential by stretching, moving and breathing at your own pace. There are no comparisons with how well other people can do the exercises. If you are doing your best, that is the best way of doing it. It is not a competition. It is not a contest. It is simply a way to feel better and better, to be happy and healthy, and to enjoy life to the fullest.

Deep within each of us lies the potential for perfection. This potential is spiritual in nature and is often blocked or displaced by the difficulties we face in life. Zen Yoga offers the opportunity to become aware of that spiritual essence and give it the nourishment it needs to grow and flourish.

Zen Yoga is not about what you **can't** do. It has been designed to be accessible to anyone regardless of their level of fitness or spiritual development. The most important challenge comes from within. Most of us are seeking more from life. Unfortunately, life itself often gets in the way of our search. Zen Yoga offers an opportunity to get to know the self…to feel happy, healthy, and alive.

Learn what your own body can and cannot do.

Learn what your body will and won't do.

Learn to accept yourself.

…and learn to love yourself.

HOW TO USE THIS BOOK

This book provides a systematic approach to Zen Yoga and is a concise manual for training. It is divided into three distinct sections, mirroring aspects of the self—mind, body, and spirit. Just as each of these aspects plays an important role within you in making up your complete being, in this book they are intricately connected and combined to create a whole.

The first section, "Mind," reflects the mental aspect of the self that needs to have things explained and put in some sort of order. Chapter one, "Eastern Philosophical Traditions," covers the various influences that have played a part in the development of Zen Yoga. The second chapter, "Zen Yoga Fundamentals," goes into detail about the basics of Zen Yoga practice.

The second section, "Body," reflects the physical self and is a step-by-step guide for practicing Zen Yoga. Divided into four chapters, the exercises are grouped according to type, based on the four pillars of Zen Yoga: breathing, moving, stretching, and relaxation. Each exercise is titled and illustrated with photos and text that detail the specific elements of the training. Don't be overwhelmed. While there are a large number of exercises for each section, it is not necessary to do every single one of them. This book is intended to assist you in self-guided practice at home. Start by choosing some of the exercises with which you are comfortable. As you continue your practice, you can add or substitute different exercises as appropriate. The most important factor is to go slowly. Some of these exercises can be challenging and it may take you a while before you are able to perform them. In addition, not every stretch or movement is right for everyone. We all have different bodies. If you encounter something you don't like or that causes you discomfort or pain, stop. Omit those exercises and move on. It is important to take responsibility for your own body. Take care to ensure your body remains an ally as you progress.

The third section, "Spirit," reflects the part of yourself that transcends this existence and seeks to open you to the vast possibilities of the universe. It is a further exploration beyond mind and body into the realm of something greater. Once the mind is calm and the body is healthy, your spiritual self is able to grow and develop. The skills included here allow you to experience this as part of your training and integrate a deeper spiritual component into your life.

Finally, the last chapter, "Zen Yoga Practice," brings the threads of the sections together and provides a structured outline for continuing your practice of Zen Yoga. By providing a format that enables you to maintain and strengthen your training, Zen Yoga will become a natural and welcome part of your life.

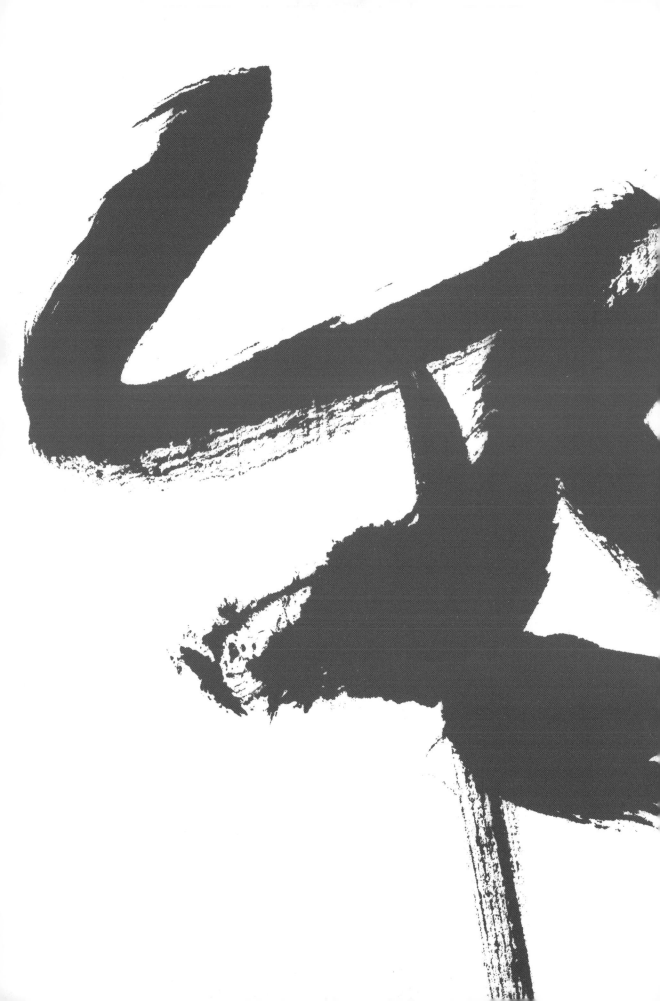

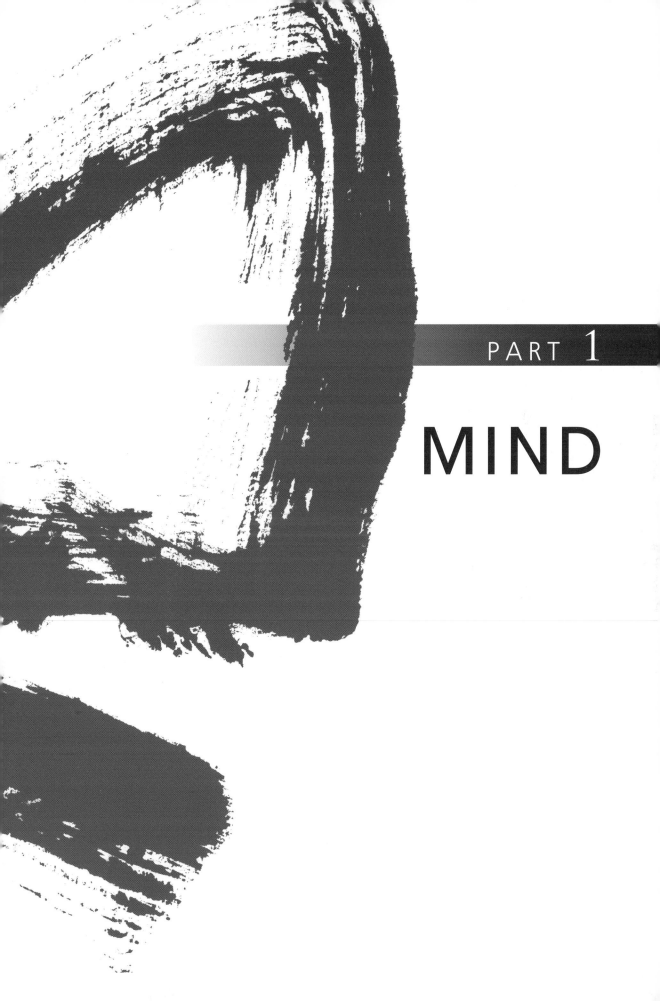

PART 1

MIND

Eastern Philosophical Traditions

Behind all things lies something vaster;
everything is but a path,
a portal, or a window opening on
something other than itself.

—Antoine de Saint-Exupery

Eastern Traditions

Do not seek to follow in the footsteps of the men of old.
Seek what they sought.

—Basho

Before beginning to delve into the actual exercises of Zen Yoga, it is important to have a general sense of the concepts and ideas that form the underlying philosophy behind many of the ancient arts. Like setting the stage for a performance, understanding some of the basic philosophy will allow you to more fully orient yourself to both identify with and internalize Zen Yoga. This will enable you to gain maximum benefit from its practice.

The philosophical traditions of the East, specifically of India, China, and Japan, represent over 5,000 years of study in the fundamental aspects of life, the universe, and our existence. While not necessarily religious in nature, they are spiritually oriented in the sense that they seek to elucidate the natural order of things and uncover the principles that allow everything to exist in harmony.

The Eastern traditions discussed here are ancient knowledge. I am not making them up. They have been studied for thousands of years. They contain both common-sense observations and deep, eternal wisdom. Consider this knowledge as preparation for your journey or, to use another analogy, the mortar that fills the space between the bricks and makes the structure of your existence a unified whole. Having that knowledge helps everything else make sense.

In the busy, modern world, we often get involved in exercise that is predominantly physical in nature. I have seen people at the gym sweating away on a treadmill or elliptical trainer while engrossed in watching television or reading a book. This seems very strange to me. There is a fundamental disconnect between the body and the mind when one trains in this manner. I will address this in a later chapter. For the moment I would simply like to say that following a practice of purely physical exercise is fine for what it is, but in order to truly achieve harmony within, you must be able to understand what you are doing at a deeper, more spiritual level.

Having some familiarity with the traditions of the East that lie at the heart of Zen Yoga will ensure that your practice addresses not only your body, but your mind and spirit as well. A deeper understanding of how you are part of the whole universe and what principles govern that relationship is necessary.

The primary philosophical traditions discussed here are the chakras, chi energy, yin and yang, the five elements, the eight limbs of yoga, and the Tao. These traditions form the underlying philosophy of Zen Yoga and can be likened to the principles of learning to drive a car. Anyone can sit down, turn the key, put a foot on the gas and begin driving immediately. But there is some obvious training needed to make sure you get where you are going.

First you need to learn the function of each pedal, knob, and button. In order to properly run the car, it is imperative that you know how the parts of it work together. Sure, you can drive around oblivious for a while, but eventually it's going to rain and you are really going to want to know where the wipers are!

Next you need to know the role gasoline plays or you won't be driving very far. It may not be necessary to understand the intricacies of fuel injection, but knowing how to fill up the tank definitely helps.

Then, before you can proceed to your destination, it becomes imperative to learn the rules of the road in order to avoid accidents. The use and meaning of traffic lights, stop signs, and passing lanes are part of the basic knowledge every driver needs.

You also need to be aware of other drivers on the road.

And, finally, you need to have a destination and, desirably, a map of how to get there.

The chakras are the sacred places of our body that you must be aware of in order to understand how your body works. They could be described as the chassis. Just as knowing the various parts of an automobile enable you to make it run better, sooner or later you will need to know how things are connected and what they do.

Chi energy is the fuel of your existence. A constant recharging of energy is just as important to the body as gasoline is to a car. It is difficult to keep going for very long with your energy reserves running on empty.

The concept of yin and yang provides the rules of the road for the universe. It can help you understand the forces that drive existence, enabling you to function more effectively in the world.

The five elements give you the knowledge of yourself as you travel and how you interact with other drivers on the road.

The eight limbs of yoga is your map.

And the Tao is the road. It is the journey. It is the destination.

If this explanation helps…good! However, don't let the driving analogy distract you. Read through the traditions in this chapter, but don't hope to decipher their total meaning immediately. They are many layers thick. Return to this chapter later, after you have a better understanding of breathing, moving, stretching, and relaxing, and you will notice how these traditions are reflected in the details of Zen Yoga practice. Once you make a connection you can begin to explore them more deeply. If one or more of them intrigues you, I encourage you by all means to pursue your own studies.

Chakras

Chakra is a Sanskrit word meaning wheel or disk and signifies the location of the seven fundamental energy centers of the body. In Western medical science, these locations also correspond to the seven endocrine glands of the body as well as the major nerve junctions. In more philosophical terms, chakras represent the various developmental stages of life as well as levels of consciousness. Each chakra can be imagined as a valve that is responsible for regulating energy flow throughout the body and is associated with a corresponding special part of it.

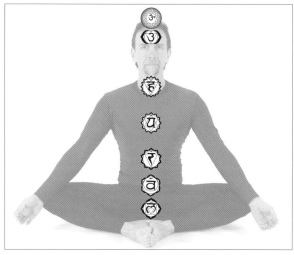

Chakras—the sacred places of the body

THE ROOT CHAKRA

The first chakra is located at the base of the spine below the sacrum bone equidistant between the pubis and the anus. It forms the foundation of our being. It is associated with the element of earth and is related to our legs and feet as well as our sense of physical grounding within the body. It is the base of our self, and therefore corresponds to physical preservation and identity. The root chakra connects to our sense of smell. In Chinese this point is called the *huyin* and is thought to work as a principal valve regulating energy flow into and out of the body. The energy within the root chakra is concerned with our health, security, and prosperity.

The root chakra

THE ABDOMINAL CHAKRA

The second chakra is located in the abdomen, roughly three finger widths below the navel, and is related to the lumbar section of the back and the reproductive organs. It is associated with the element of water and forms the basis of our emotions and sexuality. It is connected to our spiritual self and informs us of the wants and needs of the physical body. The abdominal chakra connects to our sense of taste. Known as the lower *dan tien* in Chinese and the *hara* in Japanese, this is a primary gathering point for physical energy. The energy within the abdominal chakra is concerned with our emotions, feelings, sexual appetite, and ability to accept change.

The abdominal chakra

THE SOLAR PLEXUS CHAKRA

The third chakra is located in the region of the solar plexus and is related to the main internal organs. It is associated with the element of fire and is concerned with issues of power, control, and freedom. It is related to our ego and influences the way we define who we are. The solar plexus chakra connects to our sense of sight. The energy within the solar plexus chakra is concerned with providing power to function effectively, and with coordinating action and reaction.

The solar plexus chakra

THE HEART CHAKRA

The fourth chakra is located at the center of the chest at heart level. It is related to the heart and lungs as well as the circulation of blood throughout the body. It is associated with the element of air and is primarily concerned with love, compas-

The heart chakra

sion, and interpersonal relationships. It is the place where our true self or spirit resides. The heart chakra connects to our sense of touch. Known as *kokoro* in Japanese, this point contains our emotional being. The energy within the heart chakra is concerned with our ability to love, feel compassion, and experience peace.

The throat chakra

THE THROAT CHAKRA

The fifth chakra is located in the center of the throat and is related to the shoulders, arms, hands, and the thyroid gland. It is associated with the elemental expression of sound and is primarily concerned with communication, creativity, and self-expression. From here we begin to perceive a higher reality. It is where we begin to gain awareness of our intuition. The throat chakra connects to our sense of hearing. The energy within the throat chakra is concerned with our creative identity and self-expression.

The third-eye chakra

THE THIRD-EYE CHAKRA

The sixth chakra is located at the center of the forehead above the eyes and is related to the pituitary gland as well as the carotid arteries of the neck. It is associated with the elemental expression of light and allows us to see both physically and intuitively. It is the gate through which our consciousness begins to ascend. From here we can view our spiritual self. The third-eye chakra connects to our sixth sense or extrasensory perception. According to ancient spiritual beliefs, the third eye was considered to be a window onto the mystical wonders of the universe, but as the human race became increasingly rooted in the material world, the ability to use the third eye was lost. The energy within the third-eye chakra is concerned with our perception of the whole and with enabling self-reflection.

The crown chakra

THE CROWN CHAKRA

The seventh chakra is located at the top of the skull and is related to the pineal gland, brain, and nervous system. It is associated with the elemental expression of thought and is consciousness as pure awareness. It is our connection to the greater cosmos beyond. It integrates the qualities of the other chakras and brings us spiritual awareness. The crown chakra connects directly to our spiritual essence. The energy within this chakra is concerned with knowledge, wisdom, and understanding.

Since the chakras are the sacred places within your body, cultivating a stronger connection to them allows a deeper exploration inward. Becoming aware of the flow of energy through the chakras intensifies the connection between the mind and the body. In Zen Yoga practice we seek to activate the chakras, opening them and allowing the energy to flow smoothly among them. Being aware of the chakras during Zen Yoga training will help you to more fully experience the profound connection between mind and body.

The chakras are not simply physical points within the body, they are aspects of consciousness. Everything that happens in your life begins in your consciousness. Senses, perceptions, and tensions are all manifest in the chakras. Understanding the influence of the chakras helps you to understand yourself better.

Chi Energy
The fuel of existence

Chi (pronounced *chē*) energy is at the heart of Zen Yoga, and I discuss it here because it is vitally important in understanding some of its fundamental aspects before we move on. Chi refers to the natural energy of the universe, which permeates all things. It is called *prana* in Indian yogic traditions. Chi is the vital source of energy that makes up all life, from the smallest atoms and molecules to the largest heavenly bodies in the cosmos. It is the vital life force that links us to the flow of the universe. Chi is not simply energy, it is what gives energy the power to *be* energy. This is a difficult concept to grasp. A flash of lightning is a good example of chi. The lightning itself is not the energy. The chi energy is what gives the lightning its power to flash. Chi is the power behind the outward manifestation. It moves in a natural and harmonious flow in and around all things in existence.

The first known writing about chi is in the *I Ching*, or *Book of Changes*, a kind of divining tool used by sages in ancient China for calculating the currents and changes of chi. Possibly written around 1122 B.C., the *I Ching* is certainly one of the oldest books in existence. It contains timeless wisdom about the nature of life and how the universe works.

Chi is the natural energy that exists within us. It is the vital energy of the body. It flows into us as we breathe. It is also what makes breathing possible. The ancient Chinese philosophers believed chi flowed through the body along sacred channels called meridians, which are connected to points that regulate the flow of energy. These points coordinated the flow of energy and directed the chi to the sacred places within the body. These sacred places corresponded to the chakras discussed above. Blockage or incorrect flow of chi was considered the cause of all mental and physical problems. When chi flowed strongly and unimpeded, one felt happy, healthy, and more alive.

Chi masters believe that there are two types of chi, prenatal chi and postnatal chi. Prenatal chi is the amount of chi you receive at birth from your parents. It is a limited supply and cannot be replenished. When it is gone, the life force within you is gone. Postnatal chi is energy that is obtained from the external world. It is gained from breathing, eating, drinking, and exercise. When I talk about chi in this book, I will always be referring to postnatal chi.

We need to maintain a healthy chi flow in order to keep our bodies working correctly. The ancient wise men understood that in order to maintain proper health, the first and foremost treatment must be taking care of the spirit. Proper chi flow and balance is essential to this. In Zen Yoga, the most important means of ensuring that adequate levels of chi reach all parts of the body is through qigong breathing exercises. Proper qigong breathing keeps the body healthy and vibrant through a natural vitalization process which fights off disease and illness, calms nerves, and allows clarity of thought.

Becoming aware of the chi of the universe and how you interact with it is an important step in Zen Yoga toward realizing your individuality. Cultivating it will have a profound impact on your life.

Yin and Yang

The rules of the universe

The yin and yang symbol is one of the oldest and best-known life symbols in the world, but few understand its full meaning. It represents one of the most fundamental and profound theories of ancient Taoist philosophy. At its heart are the two poles of existence, which are opposite but complementary. The light, white yang moving up blends into the dark, black yin moving down. Yin and yang are interdependent, opposing forces that flow in a natural cycle, always seeking balance. Though they are opposing forces, they are not in opposition to one another. As part of the Tao, they are merely two aspects of a single reality. Each contains the seed of the other, which is why we see a black spot of yin in the white yang and vice versa. They do not merely replace each other but actually become each other through the constant flow of the universe.

Yin represents things that are feminine, dark, cold, contracting, receptive, and passive. Yin is negative and moves down and inwards. Yang represents things that are masculine, light, hot, expansive, forceful, and active. Yang is positive and moves up and outwards.

In life all things have both aspects of yin and yang. Dark and light, cold and hot, and contraction and expansion are examples of what yin and yang represent. All things perceived in the universe can be reduced to the opposing forces of yin and yang. The opposites flow in a natural cycle, one always replacing the other. Just as the seasons cycle and create a time of heat and cold, yin and yang cycle through active and passive, dark and light, etc. Yin and yang evolved from a belief in the existence of mutually dependent opposites that cannot live without one another. This changing combination of negative and positive, dark and light, cold and hot is what keeps the world spinning.

In Zen Yoga, when relating yin and yang to our individual self, each of us must have a balance of both yin and yang to be complete. If yin and yang are balanced, life is balanced. Lack of one means an over-abundance of the other. If yin and yang are out of balance within us, we become vulnerable to any of a vast array of physical and mental malfunctions.

An understanding of the concept of yin and yang can aid you in your Zen Yoga training, allowing you to modify your behavior when certain aspects of your self fall out of balance. By being aware of these opposing forces, you can begin to make sense of some of the mysteries that confront you as you continue along your path of spiritual development.

The Five Elements
Knowledge of interconnectedness

The principle of the five primal elements is deeply embedded in Chinese philosophy and culture. They are considered as not only the five properties inherent in all things but also the five processes involved in the natural cycle of the world. Everything in existence is considered to have a relationship with the five elements. They are constantly engaged in a process of mutual interaction and change.

WOOD

Wood represents growth. Its color is blue or green and it is symbolized by the dragon. The Wood season is spring when plants are sprouting and new growth emerges. Its movement is toward increase. Wood is strong and rooted. People with strong wood energy have clear goals. They are adept at making decisions and putting them into effect. People with weak wood energy can fall under the control of anger and indecisiveness. The wood element is related to the liver and the gall bladder. The liver stores blood and regulates the smooth flow of chi, while the gallbladder stores and excretes bile. Anger is the emotion that creates imbalance within the liver, while indecisiveness can affect the gallbladder.

Typical wood traits include a systematic thought process, high morality, inner confidence, cooperativeness, and an optimistic view of life.

FIRE

Fire represents growth reaching its maximum potential. Its color is red and it is symbolized by the phoenix. The fire season is summer when everything is growing with abundance. Its movement is toward maximum increase. Fire is hot and bright. People with strong fire energy are charismatic and enjoy leadership positions. They enjoy expressing their views. People with weak fire energy are susceptible to anxiety and restlessness. The fire element is related to the heart and small intestine. The heart manages overall circulation while the small intestine is responsible for separating digested food and drink into usable and unusable parts. Anxiety can cause hypertension and palpitations of the heart. Restlessness can lead to urinary problems.

Typical fire traits include decisiveness, confidence, intelligence, original thinking, and a sense of adventure.

EARTH

Earth represents balance or neutrality. Its color is yellow and it is symbolized by a cauldron. The earth season is late summer when everything flourishes in sun-ripened fullness. Its movement rests in stability at the end of increase, before decrease begins. Earth is productive and fertile. People with strong earth energy are well grounded, nurturing, and compassionate. They make good mediators. People with weak earth energy are prone to digestive problems, diarrhea, and a general lack of clarity of thought and feeling. The earth element is related to the stomach and the spleen. The stomach starts the process of digestion, while the spleen receives and dispenses the energy from food and drink throughout the body. Digestive problems are directly related to the stomach, while diarrhea and problems associated with the lack of clear thinking are usually due to lack of proper energy disbursement by the spleen.

Typical earth traits include organization, responsibility, reliability, resourcefulness, and self-discipline.

METAL

Metal represents decline after reaching the pinnacle. Its color is white and it is symbolized by the tiger. The metal season is fall, when growth has stopped and things begin dying. Its movement is toward decrease. Metal is a conductor. People with strong metal energy are self-disciplined and well organized. They are comfortable maintaining structure in their lives. People with weak metal energy may have asthma, allergies, or frequent colds. They can also have problems with deep-seated sadness and often are affected by constipation or other bowel problems. They are often overly critical and unable to let things go. The metal element is related to the lungs and the large intestine. The lungs move vital energy throughout the body while the large intestine is responsible for receiving and discharging waste. Breathing problems, colds, and acute sadness are related to the lungs. Constipation and other bowel issues correspond to the large intestine.

Typical metal traits include ambition, determination, energy, self-reliance, and relentlessness.

WATER

Water represents decline reaching its maximum retraction. Its color is black and it is symbolized by the tortoise. The water season is winter when everything is dead or dormant. Its movement is toward maximum decrease. Water is cold and wet. People with abundant water energy are strong, fearless, and determined. They are able to persevere through hardship by relying on willpower. People with weak water energy are susceptible to urination difficulties as well as to fertility and sexuality-related problems. They can be fearful and withdrawn. The water element is related to the bladder and the kidneys. The bladder receives, stores, and excretes urine. Water metabolism dissipates fluids throughout the body, lubricating it and accumulating in the kidneys. The kidneys also gather, store, and dispense water and fluid throughout the body. Urination problems are directly related to the bladder while any issues involving sexuality or fertility come under the influence of the kidneys.

Typical water traits include intuitiveness, expressiveness, flexibility, persuasiveness, and diplomacy in interactions.

RELATIONSHIPS

Each element is intricately entwined with the others. There are two main cycles within the five elements: the promotion cycle and the controlling cycle.

Promotion Cycle

The promotion cycle is similar to the relationship a mother has with a child. The child is unable to reach its potential without nurturing from the mother.

> Wood promotes fire. Fire cannot exist without wood to burn.
> Fire promotes earth. The ashes that result from fire become earth.
> Earth promotes metal. Metal is created deep within the earth.
> Metal promotes water. Metal gives off water vapor.
> Water promotes wood. Wood cannot grow without water.

Controlling Cycle

The controlling cycle is sometimes called the destroying or conquest cycle. The relationship can be thought of as similar to an elder disciplining a child.

> Wood controls earth. Wood displaces earth as it grows.
> Earth controls water. Water flows where the earth leads.
> Water controls fire. Fire is doused by water.
> Fire controls metal. Metal is melted by fire.
> Metal controls wood. Wood is cut by metal.

Each person has some combination of the five elements within. Being aware of these elements can give you insight into why you react in certain ways to certain situations. In Zen Yoga training, it is beneficial to understand the five elements and know which are predominant within the self. In this way you can use the knowledge to your benefit when confronted with people or situations in which other elements have a strong dynamic. Readers are not expected to take the five elements and their application literally. Instead, let them be symbols of real states of body and mind, and draw from them insights into your individuality. Doing so will assist you in discovering the workings of the universe.

The Eight Limbs of Yoga

The guide

As discussed earlier in the section on yoga, any spiritual practice or discipline that helps individuals awaken and realize their connection to something larger and more profound than their individual existence can be considered a type of yoga practice. Zen Yoga is most assuredly a yoga practice.

Unfortunately, modern yoga in the West has tended to move away from the more spiritual aspects of traditional yoga and to focus predominantly on the physical realm of yoga training. Zen Yoga is concerned with maintaining the spiritual aspect of yoga training as an integral dimension of practice. Understanding the eight limbs of yoga will help you to realize that there is something much more profound than simply the act of putting your body into a position and breathing. As my yoga teacher, Shanti-ji, said many times, "Yoga is a spiritual journey, vast and profound."

Traditionally, yoga is often compared to a tree. It can be divided into eight different aspects, or limbs, which represent the various sections of learning and correspond to parts of the tree. The eight limbs are *yama, niyama, asana, pranayama, pratyahara, dharana, dhyana,* and *samadhi.* Let's look at each as they can be imagined to be parts of the tree.

YAMA

Yama represents the roots of the tree. The five abstentions of *yama* are a method of control over the self. They are the basis of our relationship to the outside world and other beings. The five abstentions are

- *Ahimsa*—nonviolence

- *Satya*—truthfulness

- *Asteya*—freedom from avarice (a desire to have wealth)

- *Brahmacharya*—control of sexual desire

- *Aparigraha*—freedom from greed

Adhering to the five abstentions keeps us centered and rooted in our true self. They keep the spirit clean.

NIYAMA

Niyama represents the trunk of the tree rising out of the ground. It comprises the five observances which lead to perception of the self. They are the basis of our relationship to our self. The five observances are

- *Saucha*—cleanliness or purity

- *Santosa*—contentment

- *Tapas*—ardor (passion)

- *Svadhyaha*—self-study

- *Isvara-pranidhana*—awareness of the divine

Practicing these five observances builds a strong sense of inner harmony and peace. They allow the spirit to grow.

ASANA

Asana represents the actual limbs that branch out from the trunk of the tree. They are the postures or body positions of yoga. It is estimated that there are more than 800,000 unique yoga postures. Some are easy and some are difficult, depending on your physical ability. Regardless of the posture you are attempting, you must learn to be comfortable with your own physical body. Only then will you be able to coordinate it with your mind to bring your whole self into harmony.

PRANAYAMA

Pranayama represents the leaves of the tree that interact with the air and draw energy into the tree. *Pranayama* is breathing. It is the method by which yoga controls the life force. There are over 100 different breathing exercises. As with *asana*, some are easy and some are difficult. Learning to coordinate the body and mind, while practicing *pranayama*, allows the life force to circulate freely.

PRATYAHARA

Pratyahara represents the bark of the tree that protects the tree from the outer world. If the mind is too attached to the outer world, we are unable to journey inward. Pratyahara draws the mind in and away from the control of the senses toward the center of our being. It is introspection.

DHARANA

Dharana represents the sap that flows throughout the tree. It can be thought of as pure concentration. It brings the scattered energies of the mind together to a single point at the center of the self. *Dharana* is meditation on the memory of who we truly are and what our purpose in this life is. It is deep contemplation of our true identity.

DHYANA

Dhyana represents the seeds of the tree ready to be carried away to grow into another tree. It brings to mind the image of duality between the tree that is and the tree that will be. *Dyhana* is meditation in a state of pure thought while being totally absorbed in the object of the meditation. It is focused awareness.

SAMADHI

Samadhi is the fruit or flower that blossoms when the mind, body, and spirit are united. It is equanimity. *Samadhi* is seeing everything alike and all as one. It is the realization of being totally connected to the whole. No longer are you a single entity existing alone in the universe. *Samadhi* is the merging with the universal spirit. It is becoming one with the universe. It is enlightenment.

The Tao

The road, the journey...the destination

Tao (pronounced *dau*) means *way* in Chinese, and involves a path of thought or life that is the essential unifying force of everything that exists in the universe. Taoism is following the way.

The *Tao-te Ching* is the earliest document in the history of Taoism. It is a perspective that emphasizes individuality, freedom, simplicity, mysticism, and naturalness. Considered one of the great philosophical works of ancient China, *Tao-te Ching* literally means "the classic of the way and its power." The book is less than 5,000 words long and, along with the *I Ching*, is one of the oldest extant written Eastern texts. Authorship of the *Tao-te Ching* is generally accredited to a man named Lao-tzu, but information about him is scarce, with only legends remaining. His name means "old master" or "wise sage." But seeking to learn more about Lao-tzu only distracts us from his teachings.

The Tao is all encompassing. Despite the appearance of differences in the world, within the Tao everything is one. Since all is one, the issues of true or false and good or evil are irrelevant, arising only when people cannot see beyond their narrow perception of reality. Taoism is a system of philosophical thought that puts emphasis on the spiritual life instead of the material world. The Tao is considered unnamed and unknowable. Followers of the Tao avoid wasting their energies on the pursuit of wealth, power, knowledge, and other distractions. Instead, they concentrate on the reality of life itself: of breathing, moving, and living in harmony with the natural world. Because all is considered one, life and death merge into each other and immortality can be achieved.

Living the way of the Tao can be expressed by the term *wu-wei*, which means "doing, not doing." This concept does not signify non-action; it hints at action without attachment to the action, action without thought of the action.

The power of the Tao lies in simplicity, and yet it teaches one to become a master of all things by learning to go with the natural flow of the universe. Trying to walk upstream against the river is pointless. It is better to accept that change is inevitable, learn to embrace it, and make the most of it when it comes.

The fundamental teachings of the Tao present basic wisdom by which to live. They are

BE CAREFUL—as if you were crossing a stream that is covered with a layer of ice. Stepping too hard on the wrong spot can lead to misfortune.

BE ALERT—as if you were a warrior entering enemy territory. Spies and traps may be hidden anywhere. Pay attention.

BE COURTEOUS—as if you were a guest. There is no reason for anger or hostility; it only clouds your judgment.

BE FLUID—as if you were melting ice. Always ready to act or react as the situation or need demands.

BE SHAPEABLE—as if you were a block of wood. The shape is pre-existing; allow yourself to be carved.

BE RECEPTIVE—as a mountain valley. Water flows down the mountain. Let things come to you. Be patient, warm, and inviting.

BE CLEAR—as a glass of water. Allow the mud of the mind to settle and see things as they truly are.

Absolute happiness comes from erasing the distinctions that separate the self and the universe. Union with the Tao is embracing a higher wisdom, freeing the mind, and expanding into the fullness of existence. The Zen aspect of Zen Yoga is about existing in the present moment and experiencing the Tao by fully embracing the whole of life and the universe.

Integration

Expect things from yourself before you can do them.

—Michael Jordan

Learning the traditions and striving to understand them is part of Zen Yoga train-ing. If you can learn to relate the people, places, and experiences in your life to these various traditions, you will start to recreate yourself as a deeper, more spiri-tual being. Opening yourself up to the possibilities these traditions hint at gives you the opportunity to explore just exactly who you are and where you are going. Eastern traditions each hint at something much deeper than what we experience in daily life. We can only begin to understand this when we learn to look within for what we seek.

It is worth meditating on this thought.

While each of these traditions may have its roots in different philosophies, each is intricately connected to the others. In Zen Yoga the ideas are intertwined. At their most fundamental point they are concerned with the same thing—discovering your spiritual nature.

Allow the traditions to run like an undercurrent through your mind as you continue to read this book. In later chapters, we explore how you can incorpo-rate their principles into your Zen Yoga training and make it something much more than a set of physical exercises. Bringing the concepts into daily life and experiencing them first hand is the best way to truly understand them.

Zen Yoga Fundamentals

The journey of a thousand miles begins
with a single step.

—Ancient saying

Fundamentals

Let's start at the very beginning, a very good place to start.

—Sound of Music

As with anything, we must start somewhere. In Zen Yoga training it is best to begin with the fundamental principles that make up the art as a whole. While at first glance they may seem overly basic or exceedingly obvious, it is vitally important that we have a complete understanding of the principles in order to fully grasp the essence of Zen Yoga. Another reason for going over these principles is that, by reinforcing them, we have the opportunity to internalize them so that we can access them instantly and intrinsically, without thought or effort.

Zen Yoga is not meant to be something that is practiced at a specific time for a set period. On the contrary, by integrating Zen Yoga into your daily life, you will be training all the time. Driving in your car, standing in line, watching television, and cooking dinner all offer opportunities for doing some sort of Zen Yoga practice. And the beauty of it is that once you get into the habit of doing Zen Yoga throughout your day, you will begin to notice subtle changes in your energy level and fitness. These changes will allow you to naturally evolve into a healthier, fitter being; you will be at peace with yourself and the world around you.

There are four fundamental principles in Zen Yoga: breathing, moving, stretching, and relaxation. Each principle is vitally important to its proper study.

Breathing

All you need to do is breathe . . .
And let everything else fall into place.

—A. H.

These days, a growing number of people are becoming concerned with their eating and drinking habits, but they pay scant attention to their breathing. Yet breathing is absolutely vital to human existence. A healthy body can survive for days or even weeks without food. Without water it can survive for about two or three days. However, without oxygen the body will die in a few minutes.

People who are truly concerned with the health and well-being of their body are missing an important opportunity if they fail to learn how to breathe properly and effectively.

On a purely intellectual level, we generally understand that breathing is the fundamental action of the physical body. It is a process that is taking place all day, everyday throughout our lives, in a continuous, nonstop rhythm. However, even though we understand this, we rarely take the time to actually notice or experience our breathing. Of course, physical exertion brings us acute awareness of our breathing as we begin puffing and panting but, for the most part, breathing is an unconscious bodily function. This is a good thing, because if you had to spend your whole day paying attention to your breathing, you would get little else done. On the other hand, unfortunately, when you become preoccupied with the events of everyday life, your breathing begins to speed up and become shallow, involving only the upper part of the chest. Generally, most people who are not conscious of their breathing habits use only the top third of their lungs. The small amount of air they do breathe in seldom reaches the bottom part of their lungs. Whatever stale air is trapped deep within rarely has a chance to be expelled. If you observe a baby breathing, you will see that it breathes deep into the diaphragm. It instinctively knows that it needs all the air it can get. As we get older, our breathing gradually becomes more shallow, until we are breathing with just the top section of our lungs. Breathing becomes labored with even the slightest exertion. The fact is that, as we grow older, we "forget" how to breathe deeply. Ask most people to take a deep breath and they immediately push out their chest and suck in their belly, ready to huff and puff like the Big Bad Wolf about to blow the house down. This is not deep breathing. It is simply an exaggerated method of inefficient, shallow breathing. It may feel good and give you a surge of energy or even a feeling of power, but it is still only filling the top of the lungs.

In Zen Yoga, by becoming more aware of how you breathe you can learn to control your breathing. Then, as you control it better, you will be able to slow it down and take longer and deeper breaths. Just the simple awareness of breathing is enough to raise your level of oxygen intake and vital energy, which lead to your feeling better. As the body starts feeling better, breathing becomes easier and fuller which, in turn, brings in even more oxygen and energy. This positive, upward spiral is created simply by breathing consciously. Your body wants to breathe more; all you have to do is let it.

Conscious awareness of your breathing allows you to access chi energy and use it effectively. It establishes a connection between the physical and mental aspects of your self. Using your breath to coordinate body and mind enables you to direct the energy along the meridians and into each of the chakras. Visualizing this process increases its benefits.

If you truly have a desire to improve your health and well-being, it is absolutely vital that you begin the process of learning how to get the most out of your breathing. The first step toward this end is to understand how the body works.

BODY SYSTEMS

Within the body the autonomic nervous system is always working to maintain normal internal functions. The autonomic nervous system comprises two systems: the sympathetic and the parasympathetic system. When we are startled or surprised, the sympathetic nervous system responds to the stimulus by increasing blood pressure and heartbeat, and by slowing the digestive process. It puts the body into fight-or-flight mode, preparing it for survival. Conversely, the parasympathetic nervous system governs resting and digestion. When the body is relaxed, the parasympathetic nervous system decreases blood pressure, allows the heartbeat to slow, and encourages the digestive process. One of the problems of today's society is that the unrelenting pace of life and the frenetic energy that is generated overstimulate the sympathetic nervous system, while the parasympathetic nervous system is not given a chance to function properly. Since the systems are equally important, it is imperative that we find a way to balance them. Proper breathing practice is the way to accomplish this.

Effective breathing techniques help to naturally regulate all the bodily systems. The intake and capacity of the lungs increase, allowing us to take in more oxygen. The more oxygen we breathe in, the more oxygen-rich blood we produce. The heart pumps oxygen- and nutrient-rich blood into the blood vessels, which carry it throughout the body, via the circulatory system, to all the internal organs and out to the extremities. After circulating and delivering oxygen to all the cells and tissue, the blood returns to the heart through the veins, flushing out the system and removing impurities and toxins that build up within the body through everyday living. The cleansed blood is brought back to the heart and we expel it through the lungs as carbon dioxide. With the next breath, the blood starts moving through the circuit again. This process takes vital energy to all areas. The better our breathing ability, the more energy we bring in and the more impurities we expel.

Proper breathing practice creates a rhythm within the body, reducing strain on the muscles of the heart and slowing down the heartbeat. The stress and tension of daily life becomes more manageable simply because we are breathing better. The rhythmic expansion and contraction of the various muscle groups used in breathing also sends the blood flowing through the muscles which helps improve muscle elasticity. Finally, the deep rhythmic expansion and contraction of the diaphragm and muscles around the lungs not only enhances their strength but massages the body's internal organs as well. Traditional Chinese medicine believes there are five organs in which chi energy is stored: the liver, heart, spleen, lungs, and kidneys. In chapter 3 we will explore breathing exercises that help stimulate each of these organs.

BASIC POSTURES

Correct body alignment is another important way of getting the most out of breathing exercises during Zen Yoga practice. When the spine is straight, the energy is able to flow freely and smoothly. It moves up and down through the meridians of the body, bringing the vital life force to all the places that need it. Incorrect posture creates blockages. Energy can become trapped in certain areas, reducing its flow. When this happens, the body becomes susceptible to disease and/or sickness.

Before beginning Zen Yoga breathing exercises, it is important to have an understanding of body alignment so that you can assume the posture best suited to your current physical condition. Basic postures can be broken down into three groups: standing, sitting, and lying down. It is useful to try different postures at different times to find those that work best for you.

Standing

Standing postures are the best overall for practicing Zen Yoga breathing exercises. The feet are positioned shoulder-width apart and turned slightly inward. The knees should not be locked. When practicing breathing exercises, locked joints create stress and cause a buildup of pressure. Rotate the pelvis forward so that the lumbar area of the spine is straight, allowing it to lengthen. The upper torso sits relaxed on the hips. The chin is slightly tucked in. If you can imagine a taut string pulling up on the crown of your head and down on your tailbone, you will get the sense of your spine elongating and allowing the chi energy to flow smoothly. Allow your arms to hang naturally.

Sitting

Sitting postures can become uncomfortable if maintained for extended periods of time because of fatigue in the muscles of the back. To help with this problem, it is useful to have the knees positioned below the line of the hips. When the knees are higher than the hips, the curve of the spine compresses the upper torso onto the lumbar area of the spine. This causes breathing to become difficult and hinders energy flow. By sitting with the knees below the hips, the upper torso sits straight and tall and the lungs have the opportunity to expand fully into the chest cavity. If necessary, to assist in keeping the hips above the knees, place a cushion or pillow under the hips to allow the knees to drop forward toward the floor.

Lying down

Lying-down postures allow maximum comfort for the body, but this can be a problem since it is easy to fall asleep if the body is tired. Nevertheless, it is much easier to relax when the whole body is evenly supported. The spine should be straight and your feet should flop apart naturally. If you have lower back problems, it can be helpful to place a small pillow under your knees to straighten the lumbar region of the spine. Try not to use a pillow for your head as this can put pressure on the neck and make the smooth flow of energy difficult. Your arms should be at your side with the palms facing up. Lying-down postures are excellent for practicing breathing exercises before getting up in the morning, or before going to sleep at night.

Once you realize the importance of breathing and understand the mechanics of it, you are ready to begin.

NATURAL BREATHING

Everyday, unconscious breathing is essentially subsistence breathing. Subsistence, by definition, means remaining in existence by maintaining the minimum necessary conditions to support life. Subsistence breathing is like a farmer scraping out a meager existence on the frozen tundra of Siberia. He may survive, but life will probably be drab, difficult, and joyless, while ill health will be a constant companion. Subsistence breathing does not bring enough oxygen and energy into the body for anything more than basic life support. There is no surplus of energy that can be tapped into when needed; in fact, subsistence breathing drains the reserves of energy in the body causing tiredness and lethargy.

Subsistence breathing takes place in the upper lungs and is very shallow. It is not necessarily wrong. It keeps you alive. And it is, in fact, the breathing method most people in the world practice today. However, if you are reading this book, maintaining the minimum necessary conditions to remain in existence is unacceptable.

Breathing takes place whether you are paying attention to it or not. This natural bodily function continues throughout life. Indeed, it is the most basic of all bodily functions. We don't need to be conscious of our breathing. Yet subsistence breathing leaves no room for error. No reserves are stored to fall back on when we encounter the inescapable stresses and strains of human existence. Without fresh energy to deal with unexpected crises, the stresses of life can easily build up into dangerous, if not disastrous, situations. One of the first things many people do in response to serious injury, illness, or stress is to restrict their breathing even more. Unfortunately, the result is a lowering of their oxygen intake just when they most need a plentiful supply.

Proper breathing skills prepare the body to better cope in times of stress or shock. Learning these skills through Zen Yoga training—before they are needed—allows them to be integrated into daily life, ready for use when the occasion demands.

Zen Yoga is about making yourself feel better in body, mind, and spirit. Conscious breathing is the first step in that journey.

The human body's natural state is one of good health. If you have the ability to give your body what it requires to remain healthy, it will do so. It really is very simple. In fact, it is so simple that people often dismiss it as inconsequential. This is unfortunate, because it is one of the most important things you can do. At the most basic level, your body needs to eat food, drink water, and breathe air to stay alive. These three activities provide the energy the body must have to exist.

Chi energy is in the essence of food, water, and air. It is the power that makes it possible for us to eat, drink, and breathe. The more of this energy within the body, the better it feels. The more smoothly energy flows throughout the body, the fewer difficulties—such as illness, injury, and disease—the body encounters. If we can learn to breathe the way the body was designed to breathe, we can provide it with the energy it needs to be healthy. The better we are breathing, the better we feel. Imagine breathing as exchanging the energy we have within the body for the energy of the universe.

Stress in modern society has a devastating effect on people's lives. Depression, illness, and other problems often have their roots in the intense or hectic lifestyle people lead today. Simple skills are needed that can assist us in reducing our own levels of stress and enable us to counteract their dysfunctional effect. These skills are the key to mental and physical fitness.

Most people do not realize how fast they breathe. Next time you are in a group of people, take a moment to notice the breathing patterns of those around you. Watch their chests rise and fall. You will probably be surprised to see how many people are engaged in rapid, shallow breathing. Some will seem almost to be panting.

Natural, conscious breathing is a method of tapping into the energy that is vital to life. When you do this, you are able to build up the body's intrinsic power. Conscious breathing opens the floodgates and encourages a continuous exchange of energy between you and the universe. As a result you do not store more energy within you, but are able to sense it more clearly, as if you were bathed in a richer, more vibrant form of it.

Conscious breathing is primarily about becoming aware of, and understanding, how your body goes through the process of inhaling and exhaling air, a process that is deceiving in its apparent simplicity. Begin noticing your natural breathing patterns. When you take a deep breath, do you puff out your chest or do you expand your lower abdomen? When you challenge your body physically, what happens? Do you start puffing and panting, or do you breathe more deeply and fully at a slower pace? Simple awareness of how you breathe lets you begin to understand how your body works. As you become more aware of your breathing, it naturally improves in quality.

The importance of this idea is so great that I ask your indulgence in repeating what I have said above. With conscious breathing your oxygen intake increases. The more oxygen you breathe in, the more energy-producing, oxygen-rich blood and its nutrients flow through your veins to purify your whole physical system. This circulating blood also collects the toxins and poisons that build up within the body as a result of everyday living and expels them as carbon dioxide. Expanded lung capacity enables you to expel even more toxins, especially those fermenting in the seldom-used lower two-thirds of your lungs. Proper breathing also liberates the energy in the food you ingest.

Harmonious rhythm — breathing better

Natural, conscious, deep breathing creates a harmonious rhythm within the body, reducing stress and strain on the muscles of the heart and slowing down the heartbeat. As we shall see below when I discuss relaxation, reducing stress and tension is a major focus of Zen Yoga training. Those of you familiar with biorhythms should not be surprised to hear that an electroencephalogram of a person practicing conscious deep breathing exercises shows a distinct synchronization of alpha waves in different parts of the brain. In other words, the longer that conscious breathing is practiced, the smoother and wider the synchronized alpha waves become and the calmer and more peaceful we feel. The stresses and tensions of daily life become more manageable simply because we are breathing more effectively.

Remember also the other benefit of conscious breathing: the rhythmic expansion and contraction of the muscles used in breathing helps the circulation of blood in the body. Increased blood flow to the body's muscles also improves muscle elasticity. In addition, the deep rhythmic expansion and contraction of the diaphragm and muscles around the lungs not only enhances their strength, but also massages the body's internal organs. This passive massaging action stimulates the flow of chi energy to the liver, kidneys, spleen, and other organs, infusing them with a fresh supply of the vital energy that keeps them healthy and functioning properly.

Finally, conscious breathing balances the influence of the five elements within the body. Stabilizing the levels of each element brings the body into balance with the natural workings of the universe and creates an atmosphere of serenity.

The regular practice of conscious breathing can bring dramatic results in a relatively short time. Paying attention to the way you breathe stimulates self-awareness, and you begin to notice how your body is feeling and reacting to the way you are living and the lifestyle choices you are making. You literally start to tune in to yourself.

As I suggested, in the beginning spend some time just observing your breathing. Is it shallow? Is it slow? Try to notice how your body feels when you are aware of it breathing. The energy of the universe is there, flowing in and out of you. If you can recognize and accept that fact, you are well on your way to greater and more healthy self-awareness.

The increased oxygen content of your expanded lungs will make you feel increasingly better. This is simply because the body will be working as it is supposed to work—and you will notice the difference. This results from the buildup of positive energy as it spreads throughout your body. As a consequence, your body will start to crave increasingly more of it, in effect reminding you to breathe. It may take some time, but when you find your body wanting to breathe deeper and prompting you to do so, you will realize you are on the upward spiral to feeling amazing.

DEEP AND LONG BREATHING

Once you have discovered the importance of proper breathing and become conscious of your breathing habits, you can begin to adapt them to your needs so as to maximize their potential. You do this through enhancing the value of each breath you take. The two qualities of breathing that are most beneficial to you here are Deep Breathing and Long Breathing. While each produces a different quality of breath, they are intricately connected and should, in reality, be seen as a single method of making the whole breathing process more effective.

Deep Breathing is simply taking more air in deeper, so that you use the full capacity of your lungs. The value of Deep Breathing cannot be overstated. Expanding the lungs to their maximum capacity makes good common sense. It brings in more oxygen and chi energy while expelling more toxins. Breathing deeper is a fundamental step to developing good Zen Yoga breathing habits.

Long Breathing is the act of slowing down the rate at which you breathe. By lengthening each breath you take, you can optimize the chi energy you are taking in, allowing it to be processed fully. Long Breathing is peaceful and relaxed, providing a natural form of stress reduction and generating a sense of peacefulness. Breathing longer is another basic step in the process of developing good Zen Yoga breathing habits.

Keep the ideas of Deep and Long Breathing in the forefront of your mind as you progress through the breathing exercises in the Zen Yoga exercises chapter. It will assist in laying the groundwork for the moving and stretching exercises that follow.

Nose breathing

In ancient times, Indian yogis and tai chi masters of China learned that breathing through the nose allowed them to concentrate the energy within the body and use it to keep the body warm and vibrant. By breathing through the nose we can generate and concentrate this energy for maximum benefit. The human body was designed for breathing through the nose and taking food and water in through the mouth. But while breathing through the mouth is easy, breathing through the nose is more difficult—and also more important when practicing Deep and Long Breathing. Naturally, there is nothing necessarily wrong with breathing through the mouth. There are times when breathing through the mouth is called for, such as when we are running at full tilt and need extra oxygen. But for the majority of your Zen Yoga practice, breathing is done through the nose. When breathing through the nose, your mouth should be closed with the tongue lightly touching the palate.

There is often a soft whooshing sound as the air enters and leaves your nose. Focusing on this sound will aid you in maintaining concentration during breathing exercises.

■ Inhalation

There are a series of defense mechanisms that prevent impurities and extremely cold air from entering the body when we breathe in through the nose. First, a screen of nose hairs traps dust and other particles that could injure the lungs were we to breathe them in through the mouth. Next, the sinus passages that are lined with mucus membranes warm up excessively cool air and trap very fine dust particles that escaped the nostril-hair screen. Finally, the sinuses and glands of the inner nose fight off any bacteria that may have slipped through the other defenses. The nose also contains the olfactory receptors that give us our sense of smell, which can detect poisonous fumes or gases that could damage our health if we were to inhale them.

■ Exhalation

It is also important to breathe out through the nose. Exhalation through the mouth can, under certain circumstances, release too much carbon dioxide and cause a condition called hyperventilation (see below). In Zen Yoga terms, it might help to think of breathing through the nose like this: the tongue on the palate acts as a circuit breaker that allows the energy to flow through you, and breathing in and out through the nose keeps the circuit closed. Imagine that, if you open your mouth to breathe out, the connection is broken and the chi energy dissipates back into the universe.

Abdominal breathing

Abdominal Breathing—conscious breathing, sometimes called belly breathing—is the core process for mastering Zen Yoga and experiencing the benefits from Deep and Long Breathing. Abdominal Breathing is about filling the lungs completely. Instead of using only the top third of the lungs, this way of breathing expands lung capacity by starting from the lowest part of the lungs and gradually filling them up from the bottom. The focus, therefore, is directed to the lower *dan tien*. I use the term *dan tien* here instead of *abdominal chakra* because in Chinese philosophy the *dan tien* corresponds to not only the abdominal chakra point on the belly, but to the whole area of the abdomen, from the navel back to the spine. This central point, deep inside the body, is where energy is gathered. It is the body's center of gravity, very close to the umbilicus where we were connected to our mothers before birth. For Zen Yoga practice you should think of this area as a ball that expands and contracts with your breath. Alternatively, you could imagine that it is a cauldron where energy is stored.

Abdominal Breathing is the practice of breathing into the *dan tien*. Of course, Western scientific minds will say that you are not actually breathing into your abdomen. What is actually happening is that the extension of the diaphragm muscles creates a vacuum that draws the lungs deeper down into the chest cavity, allowing them to expand to their maximum. Chinese philosophy, being more spiritual in nature, regards the flow of energy into the *dan tien* as just as real as the breath filling the lungs.

Whatever way you choose to view it, regular Abdominal Breathing strengthens the abdominal muscles and gives the lungs a measure of elasticity that can increase their overall capacity. It also fills the body with chi energy.

There are two methods of Abdominal Breathing: Basic Abdominal Breathing and Reverse Abdominal Breathing.

■ Basic Abdominal Breathing

Basic Abdominal Breathing is both a respiratory action and a muscular action. By focusing on the *dan tien* and using the muscles of the abdomen to push out as you breathe in, you expand the lungs fully, enabling you to take a deeper breath. Many people find this type of breathing difficult when they first start practicing it because shallow breathing has become so deeply ingrained. However, in a short time and with a little practice, they come to find this breathing much more fulfilling and beneficial as their body starts to feel better.

■ Reverse Abdominal Breathing

Reverse Abdominal Breathing is the opposite of Basic Abdominal Breathing, reversing the natural flow of the breath and thereby increasing the body's ability to generate power. Sometimes called Taoist breathing, Reverse Abdominal Breathing is practiced by martial arts students, since it strengthens the abdominal muscles and calls for focused concentration on the *dan tien* area. It is a breathing method that is especially valuable when we need immediate strength or energy. When fighting, martial arts practitioners frequently yell as they complete a strike. They are using their breathing to generate power as they execute the movement.

To practice Reverse Abdominal Breathing, inhale through the nose and slowly draw the abdomen in and up. Your upper chest will naturally expand as oxygen fills your lungs. As you inhale, feel as if you are contracting the whole abdominal area. Don't be overanxious and squeeze too forcefully. Instead, focus on maintaining a smooth and relaxed feeling within the body. When the lungs are at their maximum capacity, slowly and smoothly exhale through the nose. As you exhale, release the abdomen and push it out and down. Imagine that while the air is leaving through the nose, the vital energy is filling up the abdominal cavity. Take your time and make sure you are filling yourself to maximum capacity and emptying completely with each breath. Remember, as I mentioned above, it is both a respiratory as well as a muscular action.

While Basic Abdominal Breathing is difficult to do initially, Reverse Abdominal Breathing is more difficult to do correctly, since it requires more muscular strength and coordination in the abdomen. When first beginning to explore Zen Yoga breathing exercises, it is not recommended that you spend a lot of time practicing Reverse Abdominal Breathing. It is, however, important to know the difference and to be familiar with the principle. If you try to blow up a balloon while keeping one hand on your stomach, you will notice that your abdomen naturally expands instead of contracting during exhalation. This is also true if you try to push a heavy object, such as a car that has run out of gas. In order to effectively use the power of your breath, your stomach muscles need to expand as you push. This is Reverse Abdominal Breathing being used by the body.

Begin to practice Reverse Abdominal Breathing when you feel comfortable with the progress you've made in normal conscious breathing. Since this breathing generates power inside the body, it can almost be intoxicating at first. Take your time, and be sure to go at an easy pace. Always resume normal conscious breathing for a short period of time after practicing Reverse Abdominal Breathing.

As a general rule, Abdominal Breathing is grounding, peaceful, and helps replenish energy reserves within the body. Reverse Abdominal Breathing has more to do with the generation of power and allows you to direct the energy through the body.

Finally, remember to maintain the qualities of Deep and Long Breathing when you are engaged in Abdominal Breathing. The deeper you take the air into your lungs, the deeper the energy is able to penetrate into your being. The longer you take to perform the act of breathing, the longer the energy has in which to be processed in your body. Just being aware of these qualities will be beneficial for you.

Hyperventilation

Do not confuse conscious breathing with hyperventilation, which is sometimes called overbreathing. Hyperventilation is abnormally rapid, shallow breathing through the mouth and using only the top of the chest. It results in an excessive loss from the blood of carbon dioxide, which is what helps keep the breathing muscles functioning properly.

When the carbon dioxide and oxygen levels are not balanced, dizziness and lightheadedness are common. This is because hyperventilation causes constriction of the arteries, including the carotid artery that goes to the brain, thus reducing the flow of blood throughout the body. It also makes it more difficult for the red blood cells that do get through to release oxygen to the cells of the brain and body. When there is too little carbon dioxide, your brain and body will experience a shortage of oxygen no matter how much oxygen you may breathe into your lungs.

In contrast to hyperventilation, Zen Yoga breathing is inherently slow, deep, and relaxing. Having the correct level of carbon dioxide enables the oxygen in the blood to be released when and where it is needed. Carbon dioxide also relaxes the nervous system by helping to keep the blood vessels dilated.

Moving

No lurching . . .
Move with purpose.

—A. H.

While breathing is fundamental to life, moving is the process of applying the bene-fits of breathing to the body. Drawing in sufficient oxygenated blood is the first step. However, we need to effectively move that energized blood to the various parts of the body that need it. Circulation is the key. As I said in the previous chapter, the heart pumps oxygen- and nutrient-rich blood into the arteries, which deliver it to the cells and tissue, flushing out the old or stagnated blood and remov-ing impurities that have accumulated in the body. The smooth circulation of the blood provides energy and keeps the body clean and in working order, ensuring that the body's organs function without excessive strain or vulnerability to disease.

If breathing is the key to bringing energy into the body, physical movement is the lock that must be opened in order to process and use that energy effectively. Movement is critical to the body's proper functioning. It ensures that the vital flow continues once the energy is absorbed. The heart provides the force that drives circulation by pumping blood through the body. Movement raises the heart rate, increasing the ability of the heart to pump blood effectively. Proper distribution of blood and energy assist the organic and musculoskeletal systems to maintain them-selves. As a result, all the bodily systems are kept active and healthy.

Without movement, circulation is constricted and blood cannot flow freely and smoothly. As blood flow decreases, the amount of oxygen that reaches the extrem-ities is reduced. Stagnation occurs in these areas and they become vulnerable to injury and disease or, if already injured, they do not heal properly. The heart then starts to pump harder to compensate for lack of circulation and the lungs gasp for air. But, since the body has not been conditioned by movement to ensure that suf-ficient oxygen is taken in and circulated, the stress and strain on the heart and lungs can be draining at best and seriously damaging at worst.

The human body was designed to be used in physically demanding ways. But modern life has changed that. We live in a sedentary society in which the body's inherent need for and predisposition to movement are inhibited. Modern sci-ence and technology have intervened and introduced a vast array of labor-saving devices, drugs, and medical procedures that, by helping us survive our sedentary lifestyle, tend to obscure how essential movement is to human health. School, work, and personal interests often keep us sitting still for much of the day. We drive short distances in our cars and spend our free time in front of the televi-sion or computer screen. What this means is that we have to consciously strive to put physical activity back into our daily lives to achieve a level that is natural and healthy. The good news is that health organizations and the media are beginning to pay increasing attention to the importance of the need to move.

MOTIVATION

Most healthcare professionals recommend approximately twenty minutes of exercise three or four days a week. The problem with this is that if we are unable to set aside twenty minutes of our busy day, the first thing to get jettisoned is exercise.

In Zen Yoga I do not recommend twenty minutes of exercise three days a week. Instead I seek to have you incorporate movement completely into your life. Everyone has a daily routine: wake up, take a shower, put on clothes, eat breakfast, and go to work. You wouldn't go to work without taking a shower or putting on clothes. It is part of the requirements you have set up in order to function properly in life. Thus, if you can simply incorporate movement into your daily routine, it will soon become a natural part of who you are. This movement doesn't have to be a regimen of vigorous, sweat-inducing exercise. Five minutes in the morning is enough to start. We all waste more time than that every morning just fiddling around.

It is all about the metabolism of the body. The metabolic rate is the process of the body converting food to energy. Sedentary lifestyles encourage slow metabolic rates. But there is no way that twenty minutes of exercise three or four times a week is going to raise your metabolism effectively. How can you possibly raise your metabolic rate with only an hour and twenty minutes of exercise a week? Metabolism is a continuous process of conversion and the generation of energy. In order to raise your metabolic rate you need to be moving more often. Exercising a few times a week spikes your metabolism for that short period of time, but it quickly falls back to its regular level when you return to your sedentary ways. In order to raise your metabolic rate you need a more consistent pattern of movement in which the metabolic rate is raised gradually and then maintained at the higher rate for long periods of time. This is exactly what Zen Yoga movement is about.

Movement cannot be neglected if the body is to exist in a healthy state of being. It is each individual's responsibility to care for his or her own body. Remember, it is *your* body. No one else lives in it. It makes sense to take care of it and give it what it needs in order to move in a positive direction. Just as with breathing, once you get started you will find yourself on an upward spiral. And when that happens, you will find you are beginning to understand yourself on a deeper level. You must look within yourself to find the motivation. Your body can and will feel better if you give it a chance to do what comes naturally.

ENERGY FLOW

As we learned above, breathing brings vital energy into the body. However, it is moving that allows the circulation to distribute energy to all parts of the body. With a strong energy flow, the body's natural healing ability is strengthened. This concept is simple yet profound in its ramifications. The body has amazing powers of regeneration and healing, but it must fulfill certain requirements in order for these powers to work. Breathing and moving are the requirements that trigger the upward spiral powered by your energy flow.

Once we recognize and accept that the body needs movement to be healthy, it is possible to do something about it. We know that when we are hungry we should eat, and when we are tired we should sleep. But when our muscles get stiff or achy and our body feels sluggish, we are likely to ignore or misinterpret the message—that we need to move, to engage in something that gets the heart pumping, the muscles limbered up, and the blood flowing. In fact, our inclination often is to think just the opposite: that we need rest rather than exercise. We have the strange notion that our batteries are better recharged by doing nothing than by doing something. But you don't recharge your battery by letting it sit on the sofa watching television. Of course not; batteries are recharged by running a current of energy through them. Moving generates that energy current. The energy flowing through your body is charging your battery. Sure, there are times when the body needs to rest and recuperate, but recognizing such times can be quite difficult, especially if you allow inertia and lethargy to have a say in it.

The importance of the benefits that movement can bring to the body and to life generally cannot be overemphasized. First, you simply feel better. The heart, lungs, and blood vessels do a better job of getting oxygen to the cells in your body. Blood vessels are less likely to become narrow or clogged. Muscles, joints, and bones become stronger. The body's natural defense system grows stronger, so you are sick less often. The digestive system works better, which can help you lose weight or maintain it at a healthy level, as well as keep blood sugar levels under control. Mental health may improve because exercise relieves stress and helps you concentrate or focus your thoughts. Negative thoughts have less chance of taking hold in a mind that is feeling healthy as a result of movement. You will probably even sleep better.

The first step in starting any effective physical exercise is to prepare the body. Most exercise programs begin with a warm-up. In Zen Yoga practice, however, the warm-up is much more than simple preparation. In fact, the Zen Yoga warm-up encompasses all of the important aspects of movement and can be used as a complete exercise system in itself (see chapter 5). Once the body is warm and loose, it will most likely seek out more exercise of its own accord. The Zen Yoga warm-up is the starting point of movement from which a vista of unending possibilities will unfold before you.

ZEN YOGA WARM-UP

The first step in engaging in any effective physical exercise is to prepare for it. Preparation often has two phases: warm-up and stretching. While they may seem like the same thing, they are actually quite different. I will discuss stretching in the next section, but first we need to understand the importance of the warm-up. Warming up is the process of raising your core body temperature. A proper warm-up should get the blood flowing and raise your body temperature by one or two degrees. If you start a car on a cold day and immediately put it into gear and drive, there is a good chance you will damage the car because the engine oil has not had time to circulate through the engine block. The lack of lubrication puts unnecessary strain on the engine. Imagine your body as the car engine. Immediately jumping into a workout or exercise without a proper warm-up is an easy way to damage your body. The warm-up provides your body with the lubrication needed to prepare it effectively for the coming exercises.

The Zen Yoga warm-up is based on the essential principles of movement. We have said this before but will state it here again to underline its importance. When the body is put in motion, the circulatory system pumps fresh, clean, oxygenated blood to the parts being moved, ensuring a smooth flow of energy to all parts of the body. If you sit in front of a computer all day or "veg out" watching television all night, circulation slows down and stagnates. Bodily systems have a tendency to deteriorate without use; toxins build up and contaminate the blood. Movement, on the other hand, reverses this process, enabling the body to recycle and purify the old blood.

The Zen Yoga warm-up consists of various exercises that focus on bouncing and circling in order to work all of the joints of the body. Joints are where the energy flow can be most easily constricted. Bouncing and circling exercises shake things up a bit and allow constricted areas to loosen.

Torso

Exercises start with the torso. This area is the center of your physical being. The spinal column runs through it from the neck to the tail bone. The rib cage covers the heart, lungs, and other vital organs. A series of strong muscles along the back and around the abdomen encase the ribcage, protecting it. The surrounding muscles support the most critical parts of your body. If they are not strong and healthy, then undue pressure is put on the underlying bone structure, which causes back strain. Most back pain is a result of some kind of stress or trauma to the spinal column. By building strong and healthy back and abdominal muscles, you take the pressure off the bone structure of the spine and put it onto muscles, which are specifically designed to handle it.

Bending, twisting, and rotating are the best methods for moving the torso. Bending the torso from front to back and side to side is essential for keeping the muscles of the torso healthy. Twisting and rotating the hips keeps them lubricated and moving smoothly. Regular movement of the torso stimulates the muscles and encourages blood flow throughout the back, hips, and pelvis.

Extremities

The upper extremities are the upper arms, elbows, forearms, hands, and fingers. The lower extremities are the thighs, knees, lower legs, feet, and toes. Circulation within the extremities frequently gets blocked at the joints. We often think that difficulties in the hands or feet are isolated problems. They may, in fact, be caused by circulation being blocked in one of the joints. It is important to stimulate all the joints of the extremities with movement to encourage blood flow.

Shaking, flexing, and wiggling are the three main methods for moving the extremities. Rotating the wrists, ankles, elbows, and knees keeps the joints open and loose. Shaking the arms, legs, hands, and feet stimulates circulation and causes blood to flow to the area.

Stretching

Even if you are on the right track you will get run over
if you just sit there.

—Will Rogers

Stretching is a form of movement, but in Zen Yoga we emphasize the differences between stretching and movement because of their individual importance. Movement is about encouraging energy to flow through the body. Stretching is more concerned with directing energy flow to specific areas. After warming up, stretching is the simplest, easiest, and most intelligent place to start any activity involving movement. In Zen Yoga we work with a stretch called the Long Stretch. The Long Stretch is quite different from the mainstream practice of athletic stretching.

Athletic stretching is mainly concerned with pulling muscles in opposite directions, often with a bouncing motion, in order to loosen and warm them. It concentrates on short extensions, usually in preparation for other rigorous physical exercise encompassing a set range of motion. Athletic stretching usually focuses on specific muscle groups to be used in a specific physical activity. Other muscles in the area which may only play a supporting role in the upcoming activity are often not sufficiently stretched or are ignored altogether. This type of stretching is fine for what it is. It is not wrong. For many years, Western societies have used this type of stretching, which has resulted in striking physical achievements. But good athletic stretching concentrates only on individual muscles, not on the body as a whole.

THE LONG STRETCH

The Long Stretch is a holistic stretching practice. It is a concept that focuses on the interconnectedness of the muscles, and works to strengthen and tone them together. The principle behind moving and stretching in Zen Yoga is that the body works as a complete unit. Each muscle in the body works in harmony with the rest of the body. As you progress, you should begin to feel this completeness during the exercises. The idea of the Long Stretch is to learn to stretch in the most beneficial way possible.

The Long Stretch works to lengthen, tone, and stretch your complete musculature along an extended range of motion. Once the extension has been reached, relaxation and breathing release the tension from the muscles. Or, as I tell my students, "reach the extension then drop the tension." Finally, imagine your body becoming a lead weight and, as a result of gravity, sinking slowly into the ground. Bring your attention to your breathing and allow it to become calm and smooth.

The long in the Long Stretch not only describes the lengthening of the musculature, but also relates to the relative length of time each stretch is held. Holding the stretch for an extended period is important. As the body relaxes into the stretch, the muscles are given an opportunity to unwind and uncoil. Releasing the tension enables the muscles to gain flexibility and reach their true potential. An effective Long Stretch extends the range of the muscles at a gradual pace, helping them to grow stronger and increase their suppleness in the process.

Take your time with each stretching exercise in this book. Do not rush through them in order to do them all. It is much more beneficial to try one stretch for ten minutes than to try doing ten of them in the same amount of time. Begin by holding each stretch for a count of three and then rest. Adjust the length of time to suit your own body and comfort level but the longer the better, just as long as you are not straining.

As with most things that actually work, immediate results should not be expected. Impatience is the opposite of what we are looking for in the Long Stretch.

Take your time.

Breathe, relax.

As you progress, you will begin to see a noticeable change in your body as the energy begins to flow and it becomes more loose, flexible, and healthy.

BREATHING INTO THE STRETCH

Once you have grasped the nature and significance of the Long Stretch, you can begin to delve more deeply into how the muscles of the body function and how you maintain them in their most healthy state. This, like most aspects of Zen Yoga training, is done with the breath. Breathing into the Stretch can be practiced when doing any stretching, but is especially effective when combined with the Long Stretch.

Modern psychological theories are replete with implicit and explicit acceptance of how the mind and its mental processes can affect the physical body. Psychosomatic illnesses, altering the pulse through the use of biorhythms, and even the unexplained remission of cancers, are only a few examples of the mind controlling the body for which modern medical science has no complete explanation. The concept of Breathing into the Stretch is simply an extension of the psychological theories through the juxtaposition of breathing, physical stretching, and mental awareness.

The power of the mind is unfathomably great, and yet we only use a fraction of that power during our waking lives. It is quite often the case that if you believe you can do something, you are right. It is also true that if you believe you cannot do something, you are often right as well. Unfortunately, the mind is usually much too crowded, scattered or preoccupied for us to be able to harness its full potential. We will discuss this in more detail in the chapter on relaxation, in which we explore the subject of meditation. For now, simply be open to the possibility that, when the mind touches the body, cells respond.

Breathing into the Stretch is an exercise in using the mind to connect to the body. It is the act of visualizing the process by which the breath is taken directly into the muscles of the body. This process tones them and activates them with energy. Muscles full of energy react quicker and grow stronger. The strength from toned muscles is far more usable than that gained through weight lifting. Lifting weights builds bigger muscles, but without tone and energy the muscles are stiff and inflexible. Of course they look good, but they are not particularly functional, except at weight-lifting contests.

Instead of building bigger muscles, breathing into your stretches enables you to concentrate on lengthening, strengthening, and developing your muscles to their fullest. When you place yourself in a stretch and then focus your mind on the stretched muscles, you encourage them to respond. By controlling your breathing and concentrating your awareness on a specific muscle, your whole being becomes focused on the stretch. The mind and the body come together with breathing, which is the bridge between them.

Breathing into the Stretch is simple. With each stretch concentrate on your breathing and bring your attention to the area of the body that is being stretched. Follow your breath into your body and lead the energy to the area of the stretch. Realistically, our Western mindset tells us that we cannot breathe air into the muscles of our arms or legs; however, it is not the air we are concerned with here. We are working to direct the energy to the muscles of the body.

Remember, there is no stress or strain in this exercise. In fact the more you are able to relax, the easier it is to follow the course of your breathing.

Simply concentrate on breathing and stretching.

With each exhalation, visualize the muscle contracting and expelling any impurities that have collected. You can lightly squeeze or twitch the stretched muscle as if you were contracting and breathing out of that area, which will assist your visualization of the breath going out of the muscle.

Again, there should be no tension or strain.

Continue long, slow, deep breathing.

The Long Stretch enables the muscles to fully process and gain maximum benefit from the energy you are sending them.

PAIN

Pain is something that everyone experiences, though the threshold in some people is higher than in others. Sore and stiff muscles are a natural result when beginning any form of exercise. Proceed slowly when stretching so as not to cause any damage to the underlying bone structure. You also must learn to recognize the difference between muscle pain and skeletal pain. Muscle pain is caused by a tightness or trauma to the muscular system. Skeletal pain, on the other hand, is a result of dislocation or injury to the joints, of bone rubbing on bone, or of nerves caught between bones. Skeletal pain is sharp and severe. Should you feel this type of pain, avoid doing exercises that may exacerbate the problem and consult your physician or a chiropractor. Muscle pain tends to be a dull ache that does not involve internal damage. Muscle pain, for the most part, is subject to your own therapeutic treatment since you are able to locate it and take steps to make it feel better. You can focus more or less exactly on the muscle that is hurting.

Relaxing

Too busy to relax you say?
Complaints, excuses everyday.
Tired, weak, and too much stress,
How did your life become such a mess?

—A. H.

Modern society has showered us with an abundance of resources and all sorts of inventions and labor-saving devices designed to make life easier and give us the time to relax and enjoy ourselves. Yet, while life appears to have been made more convenient with all of these inventions, we do not seem to have gained a sense of it being easier or more peaceful. On the contrary, it often feels as if life has sped up so much that we need to use all our resources just to hang on with no time to stop and take a break. And when they do, we tend to do things such as smoke, which is extremly counterproductive to good health. Then it is back to work with more to do than we can manage. To avoid being overwhelmed, we need to extract ourselves from the overload and devote more time to relieving stress, which involves one of the core principles of Zen Yoga.

The more stressed out you become, the less productive you are no matter how many hours you work, how much coffee you drink, or how well you have convinced yourself that you work better under stress. If you are not doing anything to deal with the stress and tension, you are not maximizing your potential and you are placing your body at high risk, making it vulnerable to disease, disability, and breakdown.

TOO BUSY TO RELAX

I can't count the number of times people have told me "I'm too busy to relax." They say this as if it is a cute play on words, or something I've never heard before. Often the words are accompanied by a weak, halfhearted smile, as if the speaker really had not wanted to say them. Stress and tension can be overwhelming and will continue to build until *you* do something about *them*, or *they* do something to *you*.

Relaxing, by definition, is a slowing down of the pace at which you do things. It is taking time to let things settle and to gather the scattered aspects of yourself together. Too often, when things become overwhelming, many people's first reaction is to bottle up and close themselves off from the world. Others panic. Still others manage to take pride in being able to push on, basking in the glory of being productive while multitasking themselves into the hospital. Are you one of the many who are too stubborn to give yourself permission to relax, or take a break?

This causes a heavy drain on your resources and personal energy and can lead to serious consequences for both your physical and mental health. The longer you allow that drain to continue, the greater the chances your body or mind will begin to break down as your defenses are worn away.

If you find yourself too busy to relax, you are already on a downward spiral in which each new challenge or unexpected incident causes more stress and tension than you have the resources to handle.

TENSION

Throughout history, human beings have engaged physically with their environment to survive. Manual labor was the method of getting things done. To manage this physical burden, Mother Nature gave us immense quantities of energy and the capacity to produce even more. Until the technological revolution of the twentieth century, healthy physical activity was built into the lives of most people. In the pre-industrial age, cutting wood, harvesting food, and building shelters kept the body strong and healthy. However, all that has changed under the impact of modern technology. We create more and more comforts, while phasing out rigorous activity. Most of the things we do in an average day require very little physical effort. We sit at a desk, confined to the office all day. We drive to and from work and lounge in front of the television at night. Put simply, most of us spend most of our time doing things that require virtually no physical exercise. As a result, an excess of energy is built up within the body. This, without an outlet, has no option other than to direct its intensity at vulnerable parts of the body so that vital organs and metabolic processes begin to malfunction. Headaches, cramps, stiffness, and other aches and pains may all be symptoms of prolonged physical and mental tension which the body has been unable to release in some healthy way.

Every day, tension is gathered and deposited in various places in the body. Headaches are an obvious example. For others tension may be in the neck, shoulders, or lower back. In others, it may be in the hips, knee joints, or feet. Still others may find it affects them internally—in their gastrointestinal tract or their cardiovascular system. Since this tension is directed at places in the body where each of us is most vulnerable, it can create pockets of substantial discomfort and pain. The body, in this state, finds it difficult to function normally. We often feel as if we have lost control. The longer this situation is prolonged, the more the body begins to break down.

Worse, we often seem unable to generate the energy to do anything about it. This is unfortunate when the tension in all too many cases is the source of the aches, pains, and twinges we begin to feel as we grow older. Left unaddressed, these aches and pains easily turn into chronic illness or debilitating fatigue.

■ Body awareness

The first step in relieving tension is learning to feel the tension when it is building up in you. It is easy to block out the physical cues the body may be giving as it tries to let you know that things are not okay. Most of the time you may be concerned with all the other stuff that is going on in your life; but in the interests of experimentation, let's see if you can let that go for a moment and turn your attention inward. See if you can close your eyes and do a thorough survey of your physical body. Can you identify places that are tightened up? Can you consciously relax them?

The physical movement and stretching exercises of Zen Yoga are methods for addressing tension. They are designed to release trapped energy and bring it back into the flow. One of the primary practices in Zen Yoga is connecting the body and the mind. If you can bring your mind's attention to your physical self and become aware of what is going on inside, you will be in a much better position to deal with the tension that builds up within the body.

Then, all you need to deal with is stress.

STRESS

Most of us today realize that stress is a principal cause of many of our health problems. Even Western medicine seems finally ready to agree. And while there are many different causes of stress, the technological advances of the global economy and the intensity with which our leisure hours are filled—with sports, television, and movies—crowd in on us, creating an environment that feeds the stress.

"Stress-related" has become the new buzzword. We have stress-related diseases, stress-related illness, and stress-related behavior. What's next? Stress-related stress? Soon, I'm sure we will see a new medication on the market guaranteed to solve absolutely all your stress-related problems—or your money back (with the appropriate warning of side effects such as nausea, headaches, vomiting, blurred vision, constipation, diarrhea, and cramps, no doubt)!

Unfortunately, there is no magic pill now. The best way to deal with stress is by changing our behavior and altering the situations we put ourselves in.

Stress is created by a number of factors, many of which I have already discussed. But the interesting thing about stress is that it feeds on itself. A little bit of stress can quickly become a serious dysfunction if allowed to take hold. A good example of this is worry. We all understand that worrying is demanding and detrimental to our well-being. It takes a lot of energy to worry, causing the worrier to focus too much on it, thereby depriving other matters of needed energy. The trap is that worry is just an illusion created by your mind and has no positive benefit. No matter how much you worry about something, fretting about the outcome, or feeling stressed about the ramifications, the actual situation will in some way, large or small, be different from what you expect. Even if you are psychic, own a crystal ball, or have other powers that enable you to predict the future, you will never solve your problem by worrying, which only uses up valuable energy. And yet many people spend inordinate amounts of time worrying about all sorts of things. And once you begin worrying about something, it is hard not to start worrying about collateral issues or becoming obsessed with the fear that you haven't worried enough, haven't taken every possible development into consideration, or won't make the right decision. So you worry about it some more. This is a sure path to serious anxiety. Why waste time and suffer the anxiety of worrying about something you cannot do anything about until the time comes to deal with it?

Then there is the stress that is caused by taking on too much responsibility, which demands high-speed efficiency and productivity. You may make commitments or promises you are unable to keep. Simply put, the amount of stuff you are working on exceeds the actual time and effort you have to put into it. The further behind you fall, the more stress you generate.

There is hope, however. Once you become aware of the causes of your stress, you can begin to take positive steps to reduce the influence it has on you. The hardest thing to do is to relax when you are in its grip, but the first thing you must do is gather yourself together and approach your stress in a calm, focused manner.

■ Slow down

The first step is learning to slow down, something that most people fight against stubbornly. Yes, I know that sounds oversimplified or even insulting. You may have heard it over and over again. But if you are able to slow down for just a moment and take notice of how fast you do things, you might be in for a surprise. Do you eat quickly? Do you find yourself hurrying unnecessarily to get places? Do you drive fast? Talk fast? Think fast? Is your life based on rushing from one thing to another in the hope of eventually catching up to yourself?

When you begin to see clearly how fast you do things, notice your reactions when something gets in the way and prevents you from doing them efficiently. If you are in a hurry to get somewhere and find yourself caught in a traffic jam, stopped by a red light or stuck in a line of people, do you quickly get upset?

A major part of Zen Yoga training is learning to bypass your normal reactions and do something different. It starts when you realize that the situation is going to take as long as it's going to take, and you can either be tense, frustrated, and annoyed—or you can accept it and let go of your stress related to it. Doing something different shocks you out of your habitual patterns and presents you with opportunities for different results. First, you need to actually become aware of those moments when your stress levels are getting too high. Then, you can begin consciously easing up on the speed at which you do things. Breathing can be very helpful here. Of course, there are times when you need to rush, but see if you can distinguish between times when you really need to and times when you don't, when you are rushing just because it is a habitual lifestyle. Chances are that whatever you are hurrying to get to will still be there even if you take a few minutes longer to arrive. And you might even be able to deal with it better if you are a little calmer and centered.

PEACE AND QUIET

Being able to relax is something both the body and the mind require to function properly, yet many people have a great deal of trouble doing it. The results are seen in the increase of stress-related illness, including high blood-pressure, sleep disorders, ulcers, panic attacks, and even depression, as well as in the tension that results from the increase in anger and frustration that seems to pervade our lives and permeate our society today. Conflict, wars, and struggle run as an undercurrent beneath everything we think and do. Neither the body nor the mind is equipped to deal conclusively with these. And the result is more stress.

At the risk of oversimplification, what we really need is more peace and quiet, a time-out from all the craziness in our life and around the world. The Zen Yoga approach works because it is based on the traditional Eastern belief that coordinating the body and mind puts you in a position to reach a state of peace and quiet without sacrificing the time and energy that is so vital to continuing whatever else you are doing. The wonderful thing is that, when you are able to find that peace and quiet, your body and mind start working together naturally. You begin to feel better, think more clearly, and understand yourself at a deeper level. This coordination allows you to focus your energies in a single direction. However, in order to accomplish this, you must learn to become comfortable with silence.

External silence

One of the most striking fallacies to which people subject themselves is a belief that watching television is a way to relax. This is a great hoax that has been foisted upon us. While you may want to believe that unplugging your mind for a few hours while watching favorite shows may be a way of relieving your stress, it is actually making things worse. The constant flickering images and the assault on the senses combined with the fragmented attention span that commercial breaks cause are contributing to the stress, scattering your attention and fracturing your rhythm of thought.

But the problem is not only television. External noise has become a significant barrier to living at a slower, more natural pace. Relaxing is difficult, if not impossible, when our attention is being disrupted by the noise that assaults us continually. Yet the thought of doing something to counterbalance the noise is daunting—what can we do? Maybe the answer lies in *not* doing something, i.e., immersing ourselves in silence. In silence we are able to gather the scattered dimensions of our identity and bring them back to the center of our being. Silencing the external noise and centering the self is the first step in achieving a more encompassing state of peace and quiet.

While sound, of course, is an integral part of life, it can also be a hindrance to exploring our deeper being. Concentration is difficult when we are being bombarded with noise that diverts our attention and distracts us. Only by learning ways to manage the external noise around us can we begin to notice what is going on within us.

While many people are bothered by noise, it is interesting to find that some people are seriously disturbed by silence. They need, for example, to have the television or radio on continuously when they are by themselves. Or in a group they often talk just to fill a silence which makes them feel uncomfortable or anxious. Why is silence uncomfortable when it offers such a rich opportunity to examine your inner self and untangle your thoughts and feelings? Perhaps that is the very reason for the anxiousness. Exploring the deeper self, or suddenly being highly conscious of it, can be frightening if you are uncertain who you are. This fear can be very powerful as you plumb the deeper reaches of your being, and you may find it easier to drown out with external noise what your inner voice is saying.

But what the fear is doing is opening the path to self-discovery, to learning truths about who you are that have been obscured by the external noise. The more you explore, the more you begin to discover and identify your deeper self.

The best method for encompassing a state of peace and quiet is to seek out ways of immersing yourself in quiet environments where external noise has been cut to a minimum, allowing you to enter a true meditative state of mind.

Zen Yoga relaxation practice starts by introducing just a little more silence into daily life. This involves setting aside five or ten minutes in the morning to be totally silent. During this silent time there are no sounds—no television, no talking—just silence. Notice the feelings that emerge. Are you distracted by the multitude of thoughts that invade your mind uninvited? Do you find the whole idea pretty stupid and think you should just watch a morning talk show? But, who is telling whom what is stupid? Does one part of your mind not want the other to discover what can be heard in silence?

As you progress, turn your silent time into a habit or at least a regular routine. If the morning is too busy or noisy, try the evening. Experiment with places and postures. Plug your ears if necessary. Do what you need to do to make it a comfortable experience. Some will say that programming a period of silence in your daily life sounds pretty silly. For others it can be a little daunting. But don't get sidetracked—focus, persevere. The benefits of bringing more silence into your life are truly wonderful. You start to find space in your life: space to breathe, space to discover who you are. But you must experience it to understand it.

Use silence as a tool to help you explore your deeper self. Do not be afraid to find out more about who you really are. If you are always drowning out that which makes up your inner being, you will eventually be left with nothing but a shell. Instead, begin to experience more fully who you are and how much richer your life can be by consciously cultivating in it a new silent dimension.

Then, once you have carved some external silence out of the world around you, you can take the next step in your journey... seeking *internal silence.*

Internal silence

The next step, after identifying and beginning to master external noise, is to meet the challenge of the maddeningly incessant internal noise which afflicts our waking hours, and often our sleeping hours as well. Sometimes called the stream of consciousness in literary and academic circles, I like the simpler terms *mind babble* or *internal noise*. Internal silence, on the other hand, is a state of being in which your mind babble has been quieted and you are able to hear what goes on behind the sound of what is going on in your head. Internal noise is the sound of the mind as it maintains a never-ending babble, offering you a running commentary on your life during every hour of the day and, frequently, night. *"I'm hungry. What's this? Who's that? This pen is not blue. Where am I going? Is that a potato? I don't think this is right. Oh, look, a bird. Turn left. Wait, what was I thinking about?"* This noise is a voice that rattles on continuously, telling you what to think. It even tells you what it thinks other people are thinking and what to think about what it thinks other people are thinking! It spends hours assessing what you like and don't like. It replays songs, conversations and thoughts over and over. And…it never stops.

This mind babble is an accomplice in the creation of stress and the insinuation of tension into your body. This process can be psychologically disruptive because you don't want to consider that your mind is not under your control. And, since such a consideration is, in fact, coming from your mind, there is a real question as to just *who* exactly *is* in control. It can often drive you crazy, especially if you have no idea what to do about it. How do you fight an enemy that has infiltrated your head?

Many of the ways people use to deal with mind babble are, sadly, counterproductive. Talking, hoping your spoken words will drown out the internal ones, doesn't work. Drowning it out with music is temporary. Escaping into the television just creates more of it. Avoidance only allows it to grow stronger.

The answer lies in seeking a connection with the cleansing power of silence. It has a magical quality, when you are truly enveloped in it, which allows you to discover things about yourself that are hidden deep within. It gives you space to think about the things that truly are important and need to be thought about.

Mind babble makes mental stress much more difficult to deal with than physical tension because it is often intimately tied to your identity. Of course, problems with identity are often aggravated by other issues, making the end result of emotional conflict and inner turmoil even worse. But, without discovering this inner being—your inner self—through the peaceful beauty of inner silence, your desires, expectations, and longings easily become an unnecessary burden, and all hope of fulfilling them may be lost.

Finding internal silence can be a lifelong endeavor. However, it is a necessary part of the journey. And believe it or not, profound shifts result from the simplest of changes. You will be astonished.

Internal silence begins with meditation.

Meditation

Meditation has been practiced throughout time in all the great spiritual traditions. It is a method of achieving concentration, enhancing self-understanding, and calming the unbidden thoughts of the mind. Only when the mind is at peace are you able to truly experience relaxation.

At its core, meditation is about touching the spiritual essence that exists within you. Experiencing the joy of this essence has been called enlightenment, nirvana, finding God, or even rebirth; it reflects a deep understanding within. Your spiritual essence is not something that you create through meditation. It is already there, deep within, behind all the barriers and noise, patiently waiting for you to recognize it and allow it to grow and flourish. One does not have to be religious or even interested in religion to find value in it. Becoming more aware of your self and realizing your spiritual nature is something that transcends religion. Anyone who has explored meditation knows that it is simply a path that leads to a more expansive way of seeing the world around you and a more intense way of experiencing your deeper self.

Meditation is not easy. If you imagine your mind as a chattering monkey which is continuously talking but saying very little of significance, you will begin to understand the problem. Without an effective way to quiet the mind's yammering, it is difficult to concentrate on what the spirit has to say. It gets drowned out by the mind babble. The majority of problems such as stress, depression, obsession, and anxiety are created from thoughts that have taken control of your mind. Even though you may know these thoughts are detrimental, you believe there is nothing you can do to counter them. But that is not true. Your spirit is there, deep within, held captive by your mind. It is waiting to be liberated and given a chance to help you become your true self. Meditation is the tool that can assist your spirit in escaping its imprisonment in your mind.

Too often meditation is described as an experience in which thinking stops. This is unfortunate, because, for most people to stop thinking is impossible. When we try it, the monkey begins to chatter even louder. Attempts to stop thinking are doomed to failure and will only bring resentment and disappointment. Instead, it helps to think of meditation as expanding awareness. This expanded awareness frees the mind from focusing on one particular thing; instead, it implies being conscious of all that is happening at any given moment and being able to exist completely in that moment.

In Zen Yoga practice, meditation always begins with breathing. As we have seen, breathing has deep roots in our being. It is fundamental and automatic; the physical action of breathing is the one absolutely continuous thread that runs through life from birth to death. It is the basic process of the body and it is the one thing everyone is doing at every moment. If we are aware of our breathing, we are aware of being alive in this present moment. Concentrating the mind on breathing gives it something to focus on while pushing the monkey's chatter into the background.

The physical process of inhalation and exhalation combined with the mental awareness of breathing bring the body and mind into harmony, which is the fertile ground needed for our spiritual essence to grow into whatever it is destined to become. The mind and body working together with the breath create a connection to the spirit, drawing it out from its prison.

So at its most basic, meditation is simply sitting quietly and breathing. In fact, any practice that can get the mind to concentrate on breathing is a form of meditation. The most important thing is to enable both the body and the mind together to become focused on the same end at the same time.

During meditation, as the body and the mind breathe together, you will begin to be aware of your stillness. Stillness, in this context, does not imply rigidity. Instead it refers to a softening and quieting of the body and the mind, allowing them to settle down as they find a peaceful state.

■ Quietism

Quietism is a word I first used in my book *Perfecting Ourselves: Coordinating Body, Mind and Spirit*. It can be considered an intermediate form of meditation that can be practiced by anyone seeking to explore meditation but unsure of where or how to begin. Quietism is a state of mind that results from letting the hectic thoughts of the mind sink down, leaving the mind clear and pure. It is a state of calmness unfazed by the rapid pace of the world around you and the myriad unbidden thoughts that vie for attention. It is a state of peace and tranquility that enables you to relax and enjoy the sense of your inner and outer selves being in tune with each other.

Learning to experience Quietism teaches you the fundamental aspects of meditation while allowing your mind to continue its babbling. Quietism puts you into an environment which encourages the peace and tranquility of meditation while freeing the mind from distractions and allowing it to settle down of its own accord.

With Quietism, we let go of the distraction and just exist. (For more on Quietism see part 3.)

Whether you are new to meditation or have been practicing for years, the only thing of importance is that you do it regularly. Meditation is not something that you do just once. It should be a continuous part of your journey that will assist you in learning more about yourself. It is a tool for making your life calmer and more enjoyable, while keeping you focused on the things that are most important. It is the secret to relaxation.

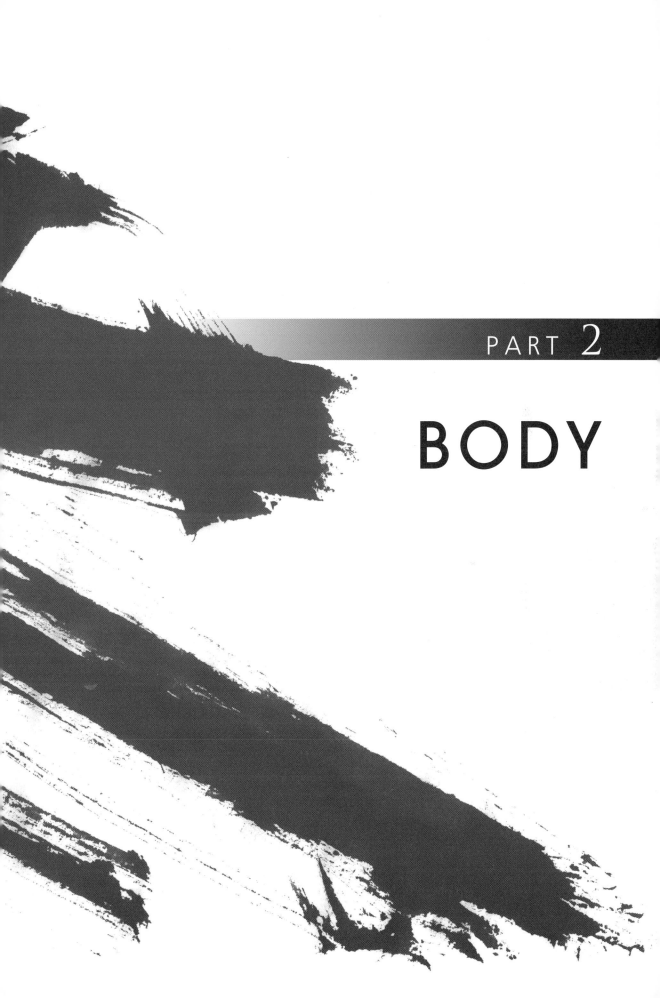

PART 2

BODY

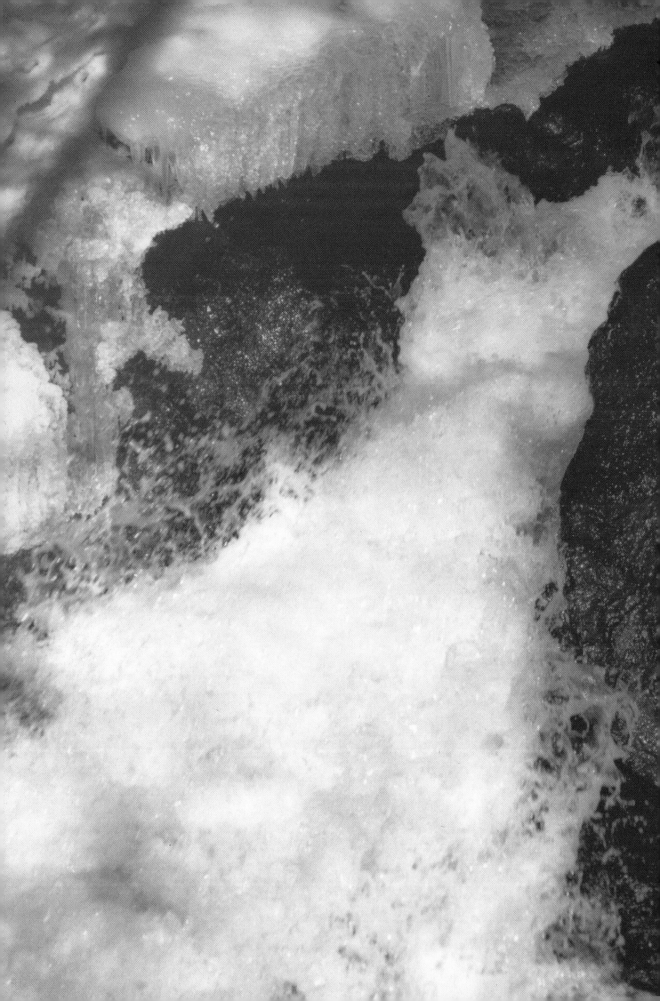

CHAPTER

3

Breathing Exercises

Teach me how to breathe,
'cause I think I've forgotten.

—Nickelback

How to Practice the Exercises

This section of the book contains the Zen Yoga exercises and reflects the importance of the physical body in overall Zen Yoga training. The exercises are grouped according to type, based on the four fundamental pillars of Zen Yoga: Breathing, Moving, Stretching, and Relaxation. When combined they create a step-by-step guide for practicing the complete art of Zen Yoga.

Each exercise has photographs and text that detail its specific elements. There are a large number of exercises here, but don't let them overwhelm you. It is not necessary to do every single one of them. The purpose here is to assist you in self-guided practice at home. Start by choosing some of the exercises with which you feel particularly comfortable. As you continue to practice, add or substitute different exercises as appropriate. But it is important to go slowly. Some of the exercises can be challenging and it may take a while until you are able to perform them. In addition, not every stretch or movement is right for everyone. If you encounter something you don't like or that causes you pain, stop. Omit that exercise and move on. It is important to take responsibility for your own body. Take care to ensure your body remains an ally as you progress.

Regular practice of these exercises will bring tangible results. Use this section as a guide and return to it as often as necessary in order to learn the proper movements and body alignment.

STANDING POSITION

For all Zen Yoga exercises, proper body alignment is extremely important. When doing any standing exercise, start from a natural stance with your feet shoulder-width apart, knees unlocked, and your hips forward and tucked under your torso. Keep your spine straight and your chin slightly tucked in.

Lying down is the position best suited to practicing breathing exercises. It allows you to relax all of your muscles and concentrate specifically on your breathing. However, there is a tendency to fall asleep if you become too relaxed or you lose focus. Keep your back straight. Allow your feet to naturally flop apart. You can place a small pillow under your knees for extra support for the lower back, if desired, but avoid using a pillow for your head as this puts pressure on the neck and impedes the natural flow of energy.

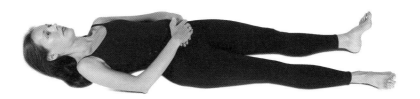

Breathing

Breathe, breathe in the air. Don't be afraid to care.

—Pink Floyd

Breathing exercises take very little time and effort, yet actually setting the time aside to do them is one of the most difficult things to do. There always seem to be so many other important things competing for your time and attention. However, there is nothing better you could be doing. Any time you spend consciously engaged in breathing exercises is like depositing money in the bank. Your body will gradually begin to store up energy and come to feel increasingly better as it is used in the way it was designed to be used.

C L E A N S I N G   B R E A T H

The Cleansing Breath is a preparatory exercise. Its purpose is to empty the lungs completely in order to allow maximum inhalation during the breathing exercises that follow. Practice the Cleansing Breath before you begin any other breathing exercises.

Breathe in deeply through the nose with a large expansion of the chest and lungs. Pause briefly and hold the breath in. Exhale through the mouth with a loud sigh, pushing all of the air out of the lungs. Continue squeezing the chest and abdominal muscles while pushing out any remaining air with an audible *ha-a-a* sound. It is usually possible to squeeze a little more out even after the lungs seem empty. Imagine that you are releasing all of the stale air and the toxins in the bottom of the lungs.

As you expel the air, relax your body by releasing the tension in your shoulders and other areas where tension builds up, such as the neck, lower back, arms, hands, legs, and feet. This will prepare the body to receive the increased flow of oxygen and energy from the breathing exercises.

THE BREATHING CYCLE

We breathe in a continuous cycle. The air comes in, circulates through the body, and then flows out. It is important to be aware of this cycle. By consciously following it, breathing becomes calmer, deeper, and more rhythmic. Breathing in and breathing out, of course, are the two main components of the breathing cycle; however, *retention* and *suspension* are also integral parts of the cycle, which are often underused.

Retention

Retention, or staying full, simply means holding your breath in. At some point or other in our lives everyone has had a chance to practice this without realizing the hidden benefit it brings. Whether it was as a child trying to hold our breath underwater or avoiding an unpleasant smell, retention comes naturally at certain times. Staying full and holding the breath is not meant to put a strain on the body and should only be practiced for short periods of time. Learning to retain the breath gives the lungs a chance to fully process the oxygen we breathe so that its vital energy can be spread throughout the body. Retaining the breath for a moment before exhaling also gives the body a chance to pause and relax before breathing out. In effect, it slows down the breathing cycle, increasing the impact and value of each breath.

Begin retention after having practiced Basic Abdominal Breathing (page 44) for a few minutes. Start by taking in a deep breath through the nose. When the lungs are completely full, stop and hold. Retain the breath for a silent count of five. If it is difficult for you to retain or suspend breathing for a count of five, begin with a count of two or three. In other words, modify the count to suit the characteristics of your own breathing patterns. When you reach five, slowly release the breath through the nose as you exhale. The exhalation should be smooth and natural. Do not collapse the lungs quickly, since that defeats the purpose of the exercise. You are trying to build up strength in the muscles surrounding the lungs. Gradual release of the air forces the muscles to actively control their contraction. A slow and smooth exhalation also relaxes the rest of the body as tension is allowed to dissipate gently.

Practicing Retention is much more than holding your breath. Pausing with your lungs full of air gives you a moment to feel the connection of your body with your mind. This process is vitally important in Zen Yoga.

Suspension

Suspension, or staying void, is the opposite of Retention. Instead of retaining the breath, the breathing cycle is stopped when all the breath has been expelled. Suspending the breath can be difficult or even feel completely alien, since the natural reaction to breathing out is to immediately breathe in. Like staying full, staying void allows the body to connect with the mind during the breathing process. In addition, it slows down your breathing cycle and assists in making each individual breath better.

When practicing Suspension it is important that you remain void for a few moments. By suspending the breath you are letting the body use up the oxygen remaining from the last inhalation. Once this is accomplished and you inhale again, the new oxygen starts filling the lungs at the lowest point, so that the breath fills them to the fullest. By suspending our breathing, we force the body to crave new oxygen, thereby assuring it is used to its maximum potential when we finally do breathe in.

To begin, after relaxing with some Basic Abdominal Breathing (page 44), exhale completely through the nose. Continue to blow out all the air in the lungs until they feel totally empty and collapsed. Stop and refrain from breathing in for a silent mental count of five (again, if necessary, start by modifying the count to suit your own breathing patterns). At first this may seem impossible, as the body's desire to inhale is very powerful, but remain calm. After the count of five, slowly begin to breathe in through the nose and fill the lungs up from the bottom in a slow and smooth inhalation. Don't panic and suck in the air too fast. By breathing in slowly and smoothly, the fresh oxygen fills the body to maximum capacity for maximum benefit. Exhale naturally.

COMPLETE-CYCLE BREATHING

Zen Yoga Complete-Cycle Breathing pulls together all we have discussed so far in this chapter into a dynamic breathing exercise that should be practiced for a short time each day. In addition to training the lungs to expand to their maximum capacity, Zen Yoga Complete-Cycle Breathing assists in cleaning and invigorating them. Practicing it regularly has the effect of naturally slowing down your unconscious breathing. Even when you are not breathing consciously, the quality of your breathing will improve. Zen Yoga Complete-Cycle Breathing maximizes oxygen intake, reduces stress, and causes oxygen-rich blood to reach the extremities in a smooth and regular flow. Regular practice expands lung capacity, slows down breathing, and makes it smoother and more even. It cleans and invigorates the lungs, and the deep rhythmic respiration of the abdominal cavity acts as an internal massage for the liver, heart, spleen, lungs, and kidneys. This passive massage strengthens and energizes them, making them less susceptible to disease and degeneration.

Of course, use common sense when trying any exercise for the first time. Begin slowly. Become responsible for your own body. Know your limits and pay attention to the feelings within.

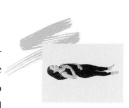

Find a quiet place where you are unlikely to be disturbed. Make yourself comfortable. This exercise is usually done in a lying-down position, though it is possible to do it sitting or standing. Whichever position you choose, be sure that there is no stress or strain on any part of your body. Place your left hand on your abdominal chakra, below your navel, and your right hand on your chest at your heart chakra.

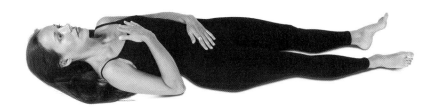

The Zen Yoga Complete-Cycle Breathing exercise is dynamic and should initially be practiced in sets of three. After each set, it is recommended that you allow the body to breathe normally for a few minutes. As with all of the Zen Yoga breathing exercises, modify the count to suit your own needs. If it seems too easy, hold it longer. Never hold the breath in or out for longer than feels comfortable. You are trying to make the body feel good. If it is uncomfortable, stop and do something different.

The exercise itself consists of four separate steps—inhalation, retention, exhalation, and suspension—repeated in a long, smooth cycle.

STEP 1: COMPLETE INHALATION

Calmly and peacefully, inhale through your nose. Expand your lower abdomen, pushing out and down as you breathe in. Once your abdomen is full, move your attention up to your ribcage and continue inhaling. When your ribcage is full, shift your attention further up in your body and expand your chest. Finally, feel your breath fill your upper body—your shoulders, collarbone, neck, and nose—to the point at which you are fully and completely expanded. Stop and hold in your breath.

STEP 2: COMPLETE RETENTION

Next, while holding in your breath, bring your attention to the fullness of your body. Feel the expansion circulating the oxygen-rich blood throughout your body. Allow your mind to follow the feeling as it moves through you. There is no set time to hold in your breath, but you may try to hold it for a count of five and adjust as necessary. The most important thing is that you are comfortable and relaxed. Don't hold your breath longer than is comfortable, but do try to hold for a moment longer than usual.

STEP 3: COMPLETE EXHALATION

When you are ready, slowly begin to exhale through your nose. Contract your lower abdomen first by pulling your belly in and up. Continue to exhale by lowering your ribcage and then your chest. Lower your shoulders, collarbone, and neck. Blow the air from your nose. Empty your body completely. Stop and hold your breath out.

STEP 4: COMPLETE SUSPENSION

With your breath out, bring your attention to the emptiness of your body. It may help to imagine an empty balloon waiting to be filled. As with Retention, don't hold your breath past the point of being comfortable but do try to hold it for a moment longer than usual. Holding the breath out can be rather daunting at first. Take care and go slowly.

A set of Complete-Cycle Breathing is three to five repetitions of all four steps depending on how comfortable you feel with the exercise. As you begin each inhalation it is very important that you don't gasp for air. Keep your body relaxed as you calmly and smoothly inhale. Start at the lowest point in the abdomen and feel the air reaching far beyond your abdomen, filling every corner of your body like an expanding balloon. Notice the sensation within your body as fresh oxygen is inhaled.

When you have completed the set, resume natural breathing. Gradually bring your attention to the feeling within your body. The changes may be very subtle at first. This is because many of us have become desensitized and divorced from our physical being. But if you are able to turn inward and observe and participate in what your body is feeling and telling you, you will begin to sense it coming to life because you are filling it with chi energy. Each time you practice the Zen Yoga Complete-Cycle Breathing exercise you will be recharging the energy reserves within your body. You will be exchanging the old stagnant chi trapped within your body for fresh powerful chi, and you will feel better than you did before.

The Zen Yoga Complete-Cycle Breathing exercise takes about five minutes if done properly. See if you can build it into your daily routine. Try to do the complete set three times per day.

Zen Yoga Breathing brings awareness to our breathing practice. When we are aware of our breathing, our body processes the energy much more effectively. Most of the time bodily functions and physical behavior are unconscious. We walk around all day, every day, rarely noticing how we feel unless there is some obvious pain. *Seldom are we consciously aware of the body actually feeling good. Feeling good shouldn't be just an absence of pain. It should be an invigorated, energetic state in which we are comfortable and happy. Zen Yoga Breathing is a way to reach that feeling.* With practice, our breathing skills will become much better and we will be able to extend that feeling.

D O U B L E   B R E A T H I N G

Double Breathing is a method of enhancing your awareness of the feeling that accompanies inhalation and exhalation. By teaching the lungs and body to become more focused on the physical act of breathing, you allow your mind to connect to the breathing process at a deeper level. The conscious effort needed to practice Double Breathing results in a noticeable coordination between body and mind. In addition, the exercise calls for a pause in each step that assists in relaxation and the release of body tension.

To begin, calmly and peacefully breathe in through the nose using Basic Abdominal Breathing. Pay attention as you fill the lungs from the bottom up. Continue to inhale, raising the ribcage and chest. Inhale until you feel roughly seventy percent full. Stop for a moment. Release any tensed-up muscles in your neck, back, and shoulders. Commence breathing in again and fill up the remaining space in the lungs. It is important to focus on the breathing process and make sure you are aware of two distinct inhalation breaths.

Next, slowly and smoothly exhale through the nose. Notice the body as you are breathing out. Feel what is happening in the bottom of your lungs and follow it to the ribcage and then the chest. Continue to exhale until you feel as if roughly seventy percent of the air is gone. Stop for a moment. Once again, relax any tense muscles in the neck, back, and shoulders. Resume exhalation and try to empty the rest of the air from the lungs. Try to release any tension in the body during the space between the breaths. It takes a little practice, but the pause between each double breath should provide you with a perfect opportunity to relax.

Breathe in. Stop. Relax. Resume breathing in.

Breathe out. Stop. Relax. Resume breathing out.

M I C R O C O S M I C O R B I T

The Microcosmic Orbit is a form of breathing meditation and energy circulation. Its purpose is to help direct the chi energy along the meridians of the body to the chakras, which serve as power centers. As the energy passes through the chakras, it grows stronger and provides a feeling of connection to your deeper self. In practicing the Microcosmic Orbit you need to open the two main channels, or meridians, on which the chakras lie. The meridian that runs up the center line of the back of the body is called the governor channel. It runs from the root chakra (at the base of your body between your legs) up the spine to the crown chakra and over the head to the third-eye chakra. The energy that runs up this channel is considered yang, or hot. The meridian along the center line in the front of the body is called the functional channel. This runs from the root chakra to the tip of the tongue. Energy that runs up this channel is thought to be yin or cold. In order to connect the two channels you must place the tip of your tongue on the roof of your mouth and breathe through your nose.

As I discussed in the section on breathing in chapter 2, the main purpose of breathing through the nose is to retain the chi energy and circulate it through your body. Breathing in through the nose takes the energy down the front of the body along the functional channel through the throat, heart, and solar plexus chakras to the abdominal chakra. The energy then continues to flow down to the root chakra and circles through the tail bone. It rises up along the governor channel, up the spine between the shoulder blades to the crown chakra. It completes the circle by coming forward to the third-eye chakra at the forehead. By keeping the tongue connected to the roof of the mouth and your mouth closed when you exhale, the chi energy is circulated back down as the carbon dioxide is released. Each inhalation brings more chi energy in and allows you to gradually build up your reserves.

Visualize the energy as it moves through your body. Bring your attention to each chakra point in succession as you move along the path of the orbit. Visualize the energy being generated there glowing with a golden light. Each of the chakra points should be visualized as being on a line down the center of the front and up the back of your body.

Microcosmic Orbit Breathing is an advanced breathing practice. It takes a long time to begin to feel any sense of the energy moving through the meridians. Patience and perseverance will be rewarded with a gradual awareness of the movement of energy through your body. Regular practice builds up your reserves, which enable you to function more effectively. The body works better and the mind thinks more clearly and allows you to create an upward spiral of positive energy.

QIGONG BREATHING

Qigong (sometimes written *chi kung*) is an ancient Chinese art of self-healing. It is a system of breathing exercises designed to assist the practitioner in learning how to understand, attract, use, and eventually master the chi energy of the universe. Qigong exercises have been studied and practiced for thousands of years.

In holistic terms, qigong is an art of energy management and healthcare using breath control. In Zen Yoga practice, qigong exercises are used to gain insight into the workings of the body and mind. Learning and practicing qigong allows you to feel the energy flowing through you and builds up your reserves. Qigong is a simple, yet profound way of breathing with your whole body and, as a result, gives you rare insight into what being truly alive feels like.

The exercises presented in this book are merely a beginning. They offer a brief introduction to Zen Yoga qigong in the hope that you can incorporate the training into your overall Zen Yoga study.

Qigong exercises usually entail moving the body as you breathe. The movements lead the breath in and out of the body. Raising the arms encourages the energy to flow to the upper body. Shifting the weight encourages the energy to flow to the lower part of the body. As your breath slows and becomes more rhythmic, your movements slow. There should be no tension in the body. Everything should feel loose, light, and flowing. As with the other exercises in this book, feel free to explore and adapt the qigong exercises to suit your fitness needs. Nothing is set in stone. Do what works for you.

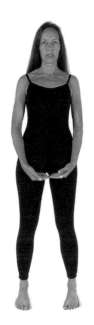
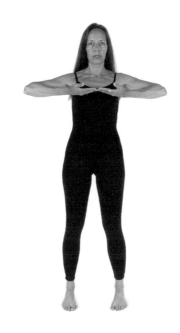

OPENING QIGONG

Opening Qigong begins from a natural position with your feet set shoulder-width apart and your arms straight down in front of you, fingertips touching. Begin to inhale and slowly raise your arms up the center line of your body. Continue lifting your arms until they are stretched, palms up, above your head and you have finished breathing in. Keep your back straight, knees unlocked, and your hips tucked under you. As you begin to exhale, open your arms out and lower them to your sides, bending your knees as you come down. Finish with your arms back down in front of you. Begin another inhalation and let the arms rise again, straightening the knees. As you begin to find the rhythm, imagine you are smoothly gliding through water, so that you experience a complete body expansion and contraction with each full breath. You should have a feeling of opening up the body, preparing it to be infused with energy.

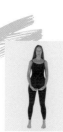

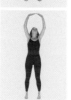

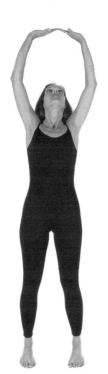
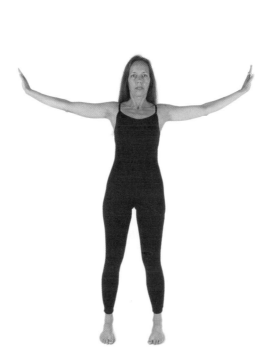

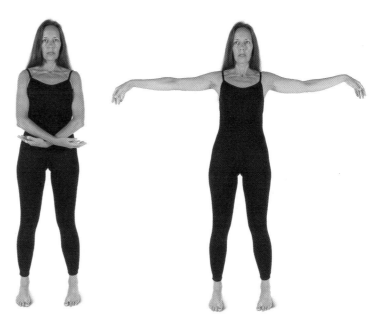

GATHERING QIGONG

Gathering Qigong is the exact opposite of Opening Qigong. It begins from the same natural position with your feet set shoulder-width apart and your arms crossed in front of you. Begin your inhalation and slowly raise your arms out to the sides and bring them up. Continue lifting your arms until they are stretched above your head and you have finished breathing in. Keep your back straight, knees unlocked, and your hips tucked under you. As you begin to exhale, bring your arms down the center line in front of you with your palms facing inwards, bending your knees as your arms come down. Finish with your arms straight down in front of you. Begin another inhalation and let the arms rise out and up again, straightening the knees. Again, as you begin to find the rhythm, imagine you are smoothly gliding through water, and experience a complete body expansion and contraction with each full breath. You should have the feeling of gathering energy and bringing it down into the center of your being.

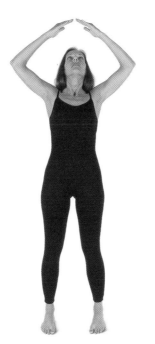

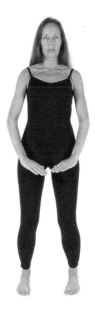

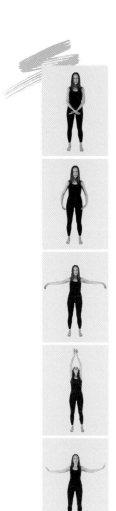

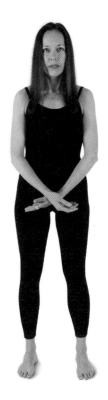

SWAN

Swan Qigong is a synthesis of Opening Qigong and Gathering Qigong. It begins from the same natural position with your feet shoulder-width apart, knees unlocked, hips tucked under you. Inhale and gently open the arms out and up away from the body. Describe this upward arc with your arms until they are stretched above your head and you have finished breathing in. As you begin your exhalation, bring your arms out and down to your sides, bending your knees as you finish exhaling. As you practice this you should feel as if you have a giant pair of wings and you are gently flapping them to the rhythm of your breath.

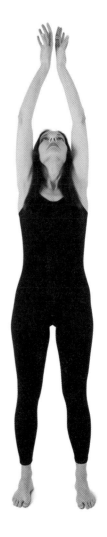

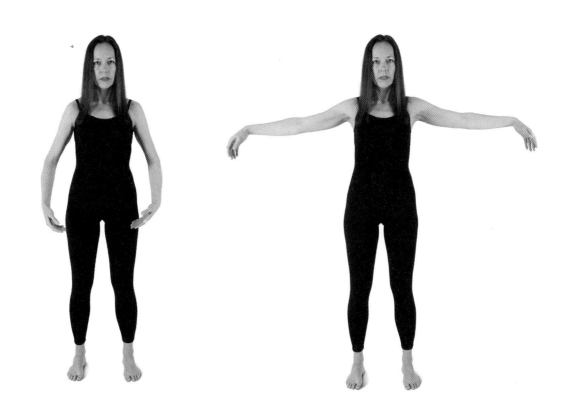

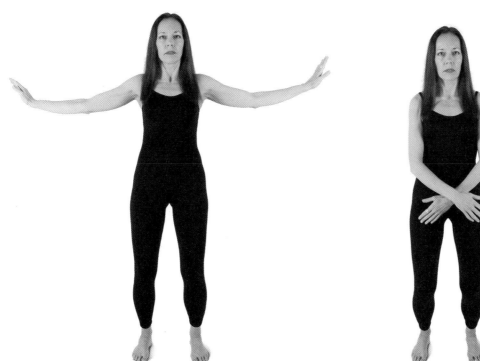

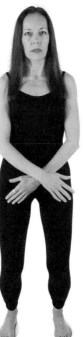

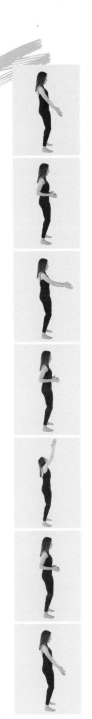

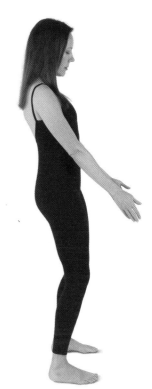

ENERGY BALL

Energy Ball Qigong is an intermediate exercise. It is especially effective after practicing the Shake Exercise in Chapter 6. From a natural position, allow the arms to hang forward in front of the body. The palms are turned toward each other as if you are grasping a circle of energy about the size of a volleyball. Close your eyes and breathe. Try to feel a connection between the center points of your hands. When you are ready, inhale and draw your hands up toward your abdominal chakra, maintaining your hand position and focusing on feeling the ball of energy. Exhale and extend your hands out to the front. Inhale again and pull your hands back to the abdominal chakra. Exhale and slowly extend your hands up over your head. Inhale and return your hands to the abdominal chakra. Exhale and lower your hands straight down to the beginning position. Repeat the whole series at least three times.

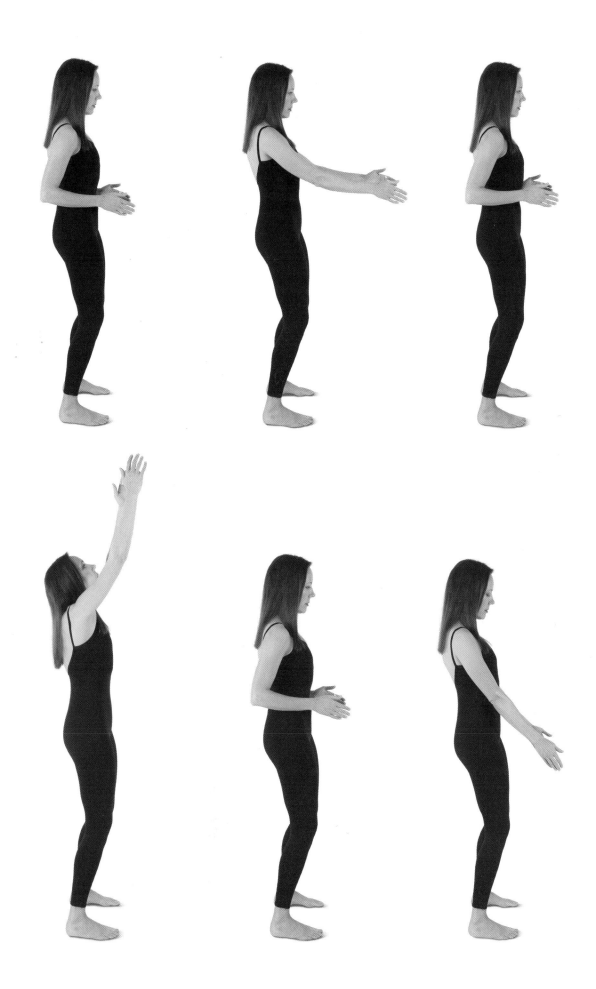

CRANE

Crane Qigong is a unique Zen Yoga exercise. It is an advanced practice that requires both leg strength and balance. It also introduces the crane fist, a hand position that can feel a little awkward when first practicing it. The Crane fist is created by bringing all the fingers together and pointing them downward as you raise your bent wrist and extend your arm.

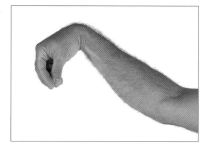

To practice Crane Qigong, begin with one leg about three foot lengths in front of the other and the feet about shoulder-width apart. Your weight is forward and your hands are forward as if pushing against an imaginary wall. Inhale, sink your weight to the back leg and raise the arms up and outwards as you form your hands into the crane fist. At the same time draw your front leg back and raise the knee up. Exhale as you replace the foot and shift the weight forward, pushing with the hands. Practice at least three times and then repeat the whole exercise with the other foot forward.

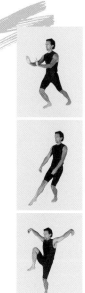

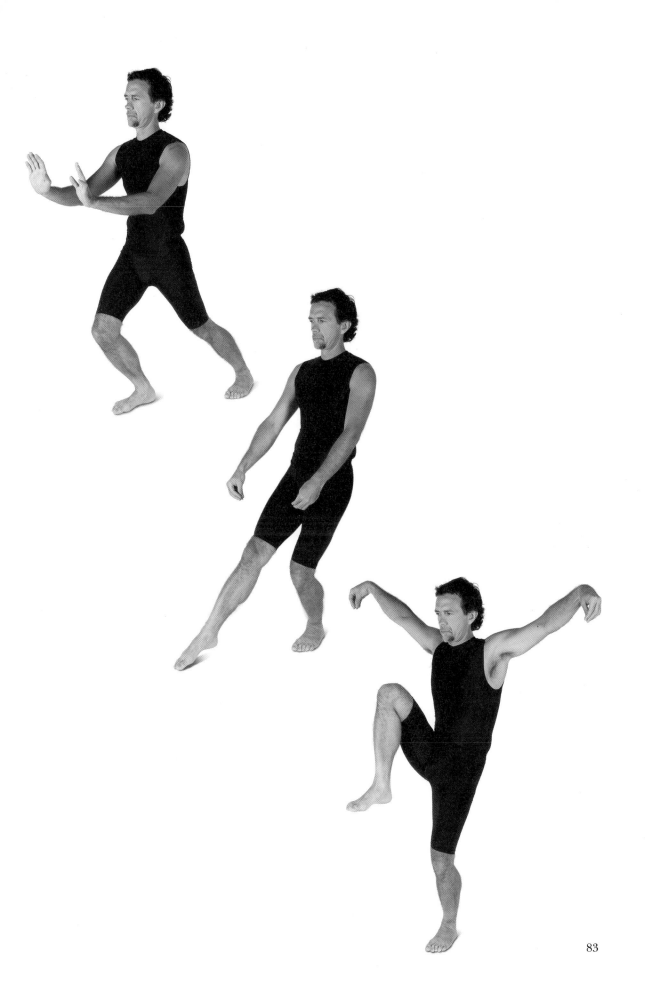

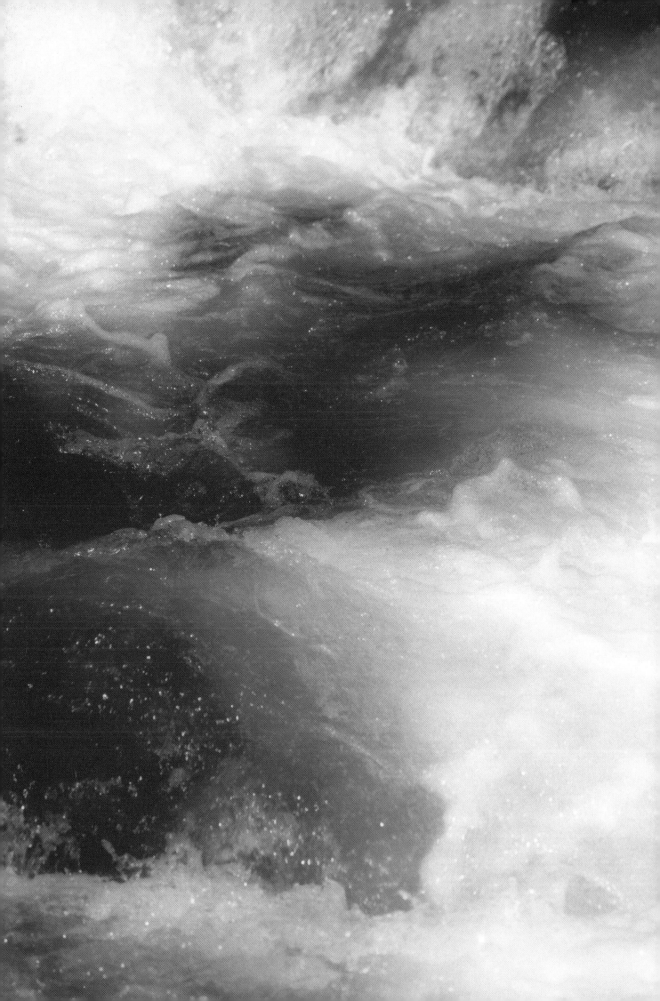

Moving
Exercises

You cannot plow a field
by turning it over in your mind.

—Unknown

Beginning

As discussed in chapter 2 on Zen Yoga fundamentals, moving exercises warm up the body. A warm-up can take anywhere from a few minutes to an hour. It all depends on how much time your body needs to get warm. Of course, the warm-up alone can be considered a full workout. The Zen Yoga warm-up exercises consist of Bouncing and Circling.

B O U N C I N G

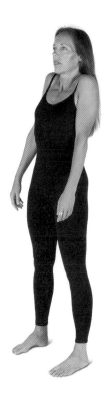

Bouncing is a way of waking up the whole body and getting it ready for the stretching exercises that are to come. Bouncing exercises are simple and easy to do at any time. It is a pleasant way to get your body moving and your blood flowing. Experiment with your breathing while doing the bouncing exercises. Exhaling as you come down assists in releasing tension.

Bouncing is done from a standing position and has four aspects. Begin with the first two shrugging exercises and then, when ready, gradually move into the other, more vigorous bouncing exercises. *For each of these exercises start with five repetitions and adjust to suit your body.* Only practice bouncing to the level that feels comfortable.

SHOULDER SHRUG

From a relaxed standing position, raise your shoulders up in a simple shrug and then drop them. Repeat this in a smooth and continuous motion, up and down. Loosen your shoulder muscles. There should be no tension in your arms, which should wiggle loosely around you as you shrug. Continue for about ten shrugs. This will release the stress and tension that builds up in your shoulders and neck, and allow better circulation to the brain.

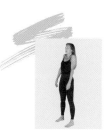

BODY SHRUG

Begin the transition to the Body Shrug after you have done the shoulder shrug five times and feel comfortable with it. Gradually begin bending the knees each time your shoulders come down and straighten them as your shoulders go up. Start to feel your whole body becoming involved in the shrugging movement up and down. The hips and legs should remain loose and light. Imagine that each time you come down you are shaking loose all the stiff and encrusted places within your body. Repeat this five to ten times.

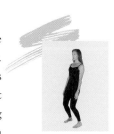

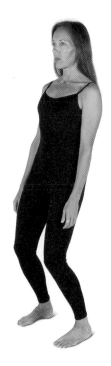

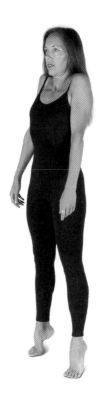

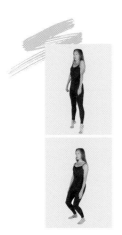

JOLT

Transition from the Body Shrug to the Jolt by starting to raise the heels of your feet each time your shoulders go up, rising on the balls of your feet, and then bouncing back down lightly on your heels when you release. There is a subtle jolt each time your heels hit the floor and that jolt travels up your entire body. Imagine it stirring up all the stagnant areas of your body and getting you ready to move. You will begin to feel increasingly loose and relaxed. Repeat five to ten times.

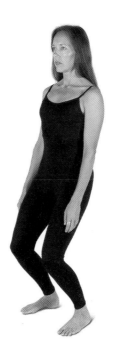

FULL BOUNCE

Transition from the Jolt by beginning to bounce a little higher each time. As you rise up, start to lift the balls of your feet a little more off the floor each time. Come down on the feet and bend the knees. Instead of jolting, gently drop back to the ground with little or no impact, touching first with the balls of the feet and then the heels. Allow the knees to bend as you complete the motion. Remember to keep yourself feeling loose and light during this exercise. At no time should you feel you are straining any part of your body. Depending on your level of fitness, try to lift off the floor increasingly higher with each bounce. Be sure to maintain the relaxed feeling.

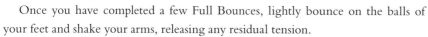

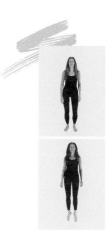

Once you have completed a few Full Bounces, lightly bounce on the balls of your feet and shake your arms, releasing any residual tension.

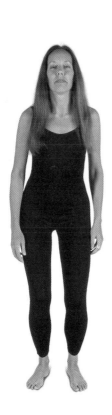

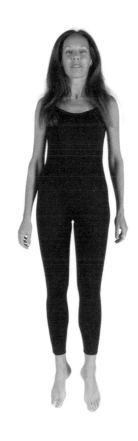

Circling is designed to loosen your joints, enabling the blood to flow smoothly and without obstruction. Circling exercises lubricate the entire joint being exercised with synovial fluid, the body's natural lubricant. Joints often stiffen up because of poor circulation, and this lubrication allows them to function more smoothly and easily. Of course breathing is very important when practicing Circling. Linking your breathing to the body movement keeps you aware and present during the exercise. Once you are doing the exercise properly, return your attention to your breath and focus on it. This mind-body connection is a fundamental aspect of Zen Yoga.

The exercises begin with the torso before moving to the extremities. For each of these exercises start with five repetitions and adjust to suit your body.

HIP ROTATION

■ Normal

This exercise loosens the hip sockets. Stand with legs apart and place your hands on your hips. Begin to rotate your hips in a smooth circular motion as if you were using a Hula Hoop. Move slowly and gently until you become used to the motion. Continue for five or ten rotations and then reverse and rotate in the opposite direction. Once your body is comfortable with the motion, concentrate on breathing deeper.

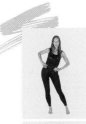

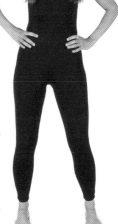

■ Isolated

This exercise brings more focus to the hip sockets. Keeping your shoulders and knees straight, try to isolate your hip joints and rotate your hips as if you were belly dancing. This is more difficult since many people have stiff hips: however, you will find that they loosen up with a little practice. Return your focus to your breathing once you are rotating.

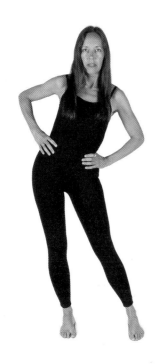

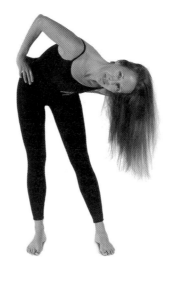

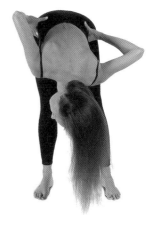

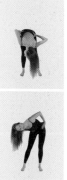
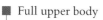

■ Full upper body

This is the best exercise for working all the hip joints. Start by rotating the hips but begin to lean your upper body into the rotation circle so that your upper torso makes a larger circular motion. Bend forward almost to the knees and then up along the side of the body, leaning back and looking up, and then down to the other side. Continue for five rotations in each direction. Practice long, slow breaths as you move.

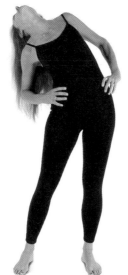

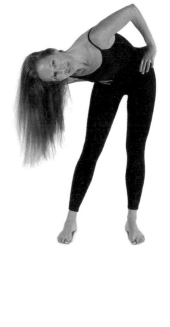

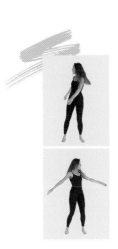

■ Twist

In contrast to the other rotation movements, this exercise is about moving the hips in a swiveling motion. Begin with legs about shoulder-width apart and the knees slightly bent. Swivel the hips to one side, allowing the arms to follow. Immediately twist the hips back to the other side, letting the arms swing freely. Continue the motion at least ten times. There should be no tension in the arms as they flop around the body. This exercise loosens stiffness and relaxes the body. Don't worry about breathing for this exercise, just breathe naturally.

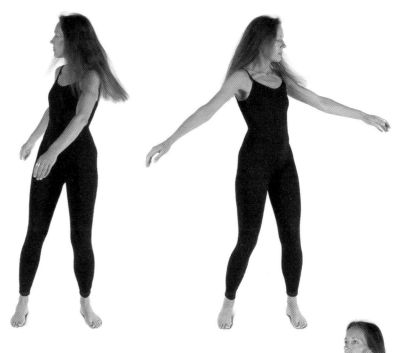

ARM ROTATION

■ Shoulders

Standing with legs shoulder-width apart, relax and begin by circling the shoulders. This is a different motion from the Shrug in the bouncing exercise. In that exercise we were moving the shoulders up and down in order to isolate the joints. In this exercise try to concentrate on making as large a circular motion as possible, first forward and then backward. Breathe slowly and smoothly.

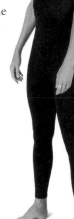

■ Arms

This exercise works on the shoulder joints and nearby musculature. Drop the arms down to your sides. Lengthen one arm and slowly describe an arc up past the ear, then back, around and down. Keep the arm straight and move it in a long, smooth circular motion. Circle five times in one direction and then reverse. Go slowly and match your breathing to the movement so that you inhale as your arm goes up and exhale as it comes down. Repeat with the other arm. Next, circle one arm and then the other as if you were doing the backstroke while swimming. Continue this motion for five rotations and then change directions so that your arms are coming forward.

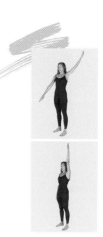

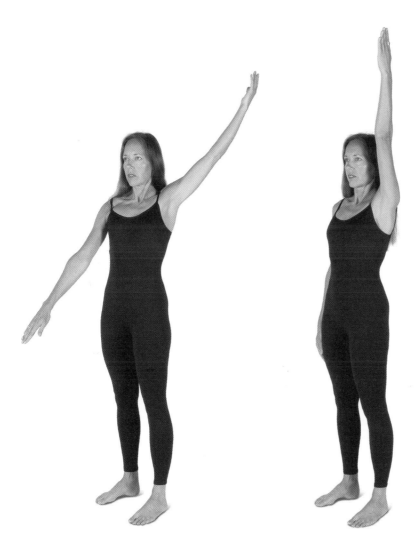

Pinwheel

A more advanced version of arm circling involves moving the arms simultaneously in opposite directions. Start with both arms extended above your head. Move one arm forward and down while moving the other back and down. The key is to rotate your hips in the direction of the arm that is going backwards as the arms reach the apex of the circle above your head and then the other way as they reach the bottom. This exercise can be a challenge, but is a good exercise for learning to coordinate the mind and body. It may take some practice. Don't worry too much about your breathing for this exercise.

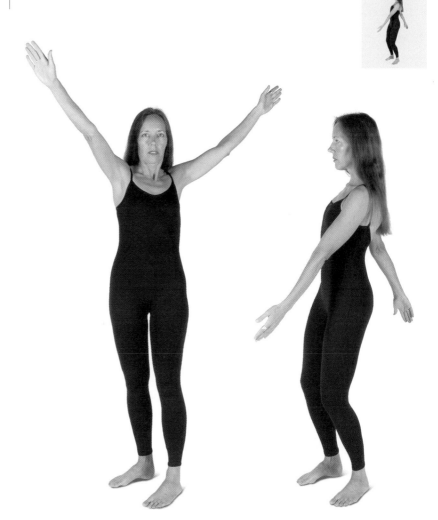

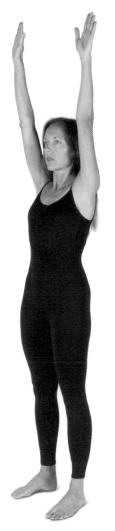

■ Elbows

This exercise isolates the elbow joints. Bring your arms up, palms facing down in front of your chest with your fingertips almost touching. Focus on your lower arms from the hand to the elbow joint. Rotate both arms from the elbow joint at the same time. Reverse and repeat in the other direction. Keep your elbows high and make sure the movement is horizontal. Repeat the motion five times in each direction. Remember to breathe once you get comfortable with the exercise.

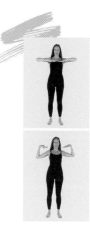

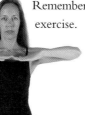

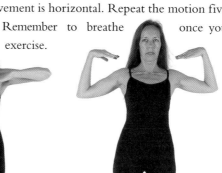

LEG ROTATION

■ Hip and leg

Next, from a standing position, put your weight on your right foot and lift the left foot off the ground. Bend your knee and bring it up, rotate it out to the side, and then down describing a complete circle. Rotate the whole leg like this three times in one direction and then reverse. The aim of this exercise is to isolate and circle the ball joint that connects the leg to the hip. Repeat five times and then do the same with the other leg. This exercise can also be done with the leg straight. Breathe slowly and smoothly, don't rush.

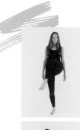

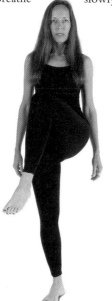

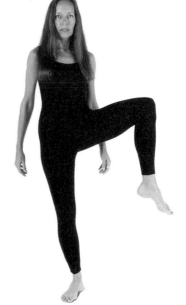

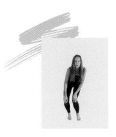

■ Knees

This exercise focuses on the knee joints. From a standing position, bend at the waist and put your hands on your knees. Bend the knees and slowly begin to rotate them in a circular motion. Do not try to push them further out than they go naturally. Always remember you are trying to make your body feel better. If it hurts, stop. Rotate five times in each direction. Breathe naturally.

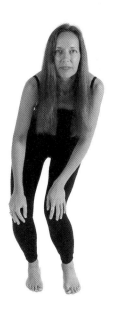

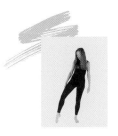

■ Ankles

This exercise loosens the ankle joints. From a standing position, put your weight on your left foot and gently touch the big toe of your right foot to the floor. Focus on the ankle joint and circle it five times in each direction. Repeat with the other foot. Breathe naturally.

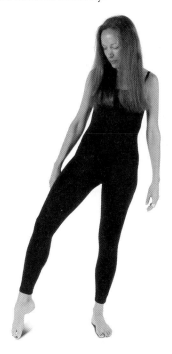

NECK ROTATION

Stretching the neck is a complicated proposition. Consult your physician before commencing any neck exercises. There are many delicate bones and joints in the neck that are easily injured. At the same time, the neck is a central focus for tension and stress, the relief of which can be very beneficial. Always keep your motions slow and controlled when stretching your neck to avoid pain or injury. This series of exercises is called Neck Circling, although there is no rotation motion involved. Rather the set of four stretches accomplishes the goal of rotation without the stress of movement that can damage the neck. These neck stretches are simple, effective, and nonstressful.

■ Front
From a standing or sitting position, breathe in deeply through the nose. Exhale and slowly bend your head forward until your chin touches your chest. On the next inhalation raise your head back up to the normal position. Repeat five times. On the fifth repetition, stop with your chin down, just touching your chest. Clasp your hands together behind your head and gently apply a very slight pressure downward to stretch the back of your neck.

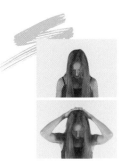

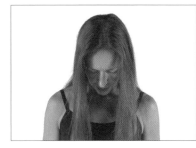
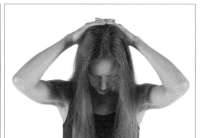

■ Back
From the same natural standing or sitting position breathe in. Exhale and slowly arc your head back so your chin is pointing up. Inhale and bring your head back up to the starting position. Repeat five times. On the fifth repetition, stop with your head back and your chin pointing up. Place the palms of your hands on your forehead and apply a slight pressure backward to stretch the front of your neck.

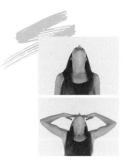

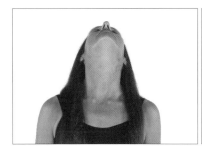
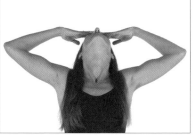

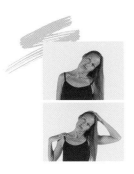

Side bend

Again, from the same natural standing or sitting position, inhale. Exhale and slowly bend your head to one side and bring your ear close to your shoulder. Inhale and return your head to the starting position. Repeat five times. On the fifth repetition, stop with your ear near your shoulder. Bring your arm up and gently rest it on top of your head, applying a slight downward pressure. Take your other hand and put it on the opposite shoulder and gently pull it away from your head. Repeat the whole exercise in the other direction while continuing to breathe in the same manner.

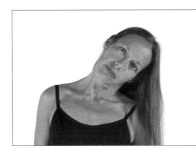 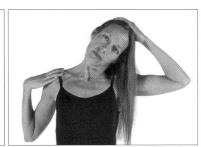

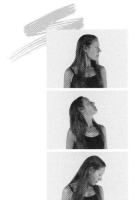

Side turn

Start from the same natural standing or sitting position of your choice, inhale. Exhale and slowly turn your head to the side. Inhale and return your head to the starting position. Repeat five times. On the fifth repetition stop with your head to the side. Begin to nod the head up and down. Repeat on the other side.

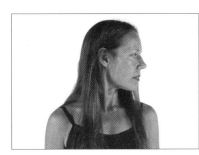 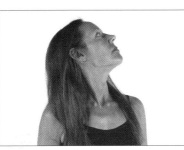 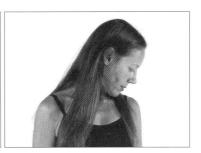

After a session of Bouncing and Circling, your body should feel sufficiently warmed up and ready to begin some stretching exercises.

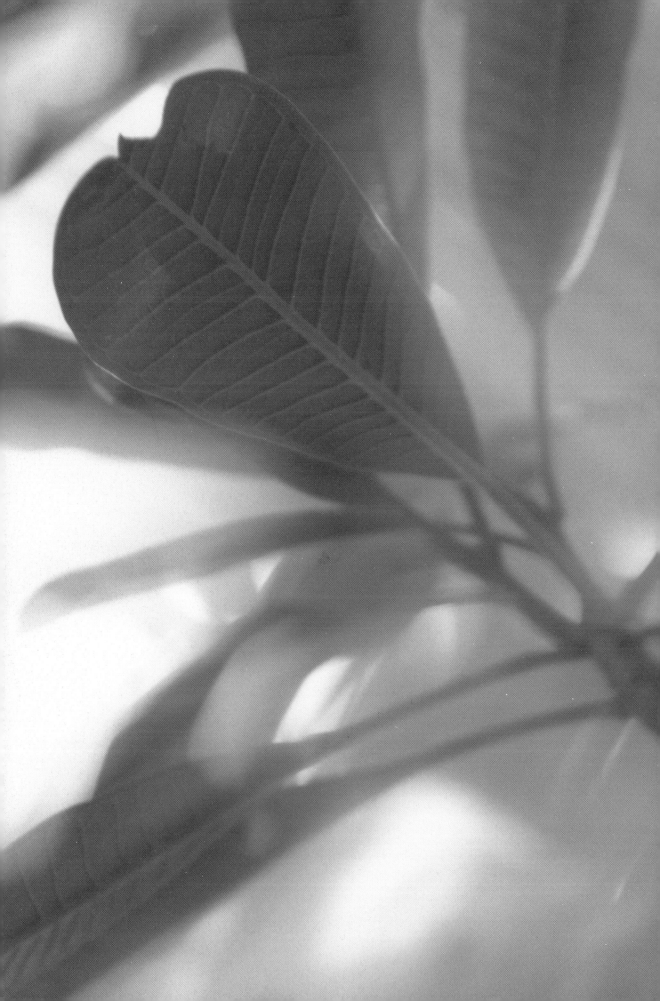

Stretching Exercises

We cannot seek or attain health,
wealth, learning, justice, or kindness in general.
Action is always specific, concrete,
individualized, and unique.

—Benjamin Jowett

How to Practice the Exercises

Proper stretching is a critical element of Zen Yoga. Incorporating some of these exercises as a regular routine into your daily life can be immensely beneficial. A few minutes of moving, stretching, and deep breathing each day enlivens the body and taps into hidden reserves of energy. Let your body experience it.

P R E P A R A T I O N

1. It is best to perform these exercises on an empty stomach. Stretching when you are full can be uncomfortable.

2. Use the bathroom before starting. A full bladder restricts breathing.

3. Wear loose-fitting clothing to allow ease of breathing and smooth, unconstricted blood flow.

4. Put on some relaxing background music.

5. Spend a few moments lying in silence before beginning the exercises.

B R E A T H I N G

I repeat this over and over, but breathing truly is the most important dimension of Zen Yoga. It is your number one priority. It is better to do half a stretch while breathing than to try and do a full stretch without breathing. Integrating breathing into your stretching exercises allows your body to maximize the energy and use it effectively. *Begin with simple conscious breathing, holding each posture for at least three breaths (inhalation + exhalation = 1 breath).* Holding each posture for three breaths gives the body time to relax into the stretch. As you become more adept, lengthen the breaths and see if you can incorporate the Zen Yoga Complete-Cycle Breathing (page 71) into the postures.

When beginning to practice the exercises use Basic Abdominal Breathing (page 44). Once you are comfortable, feel free to experiment with Reverse Abdominal Breathing and take note of the different feeling within your body.

E X E C U T I O N

Never hurry when performing stretching exercises. Rushing through stretches reflects impatience in the mind. It also risks injury. Quick jerking or twisting motions can damage the muscles and tendons. Forcing muscles and joints to respond can also lead to injury. Do not rush. Go slowly and relax as you become more aware of your body. Most of all, respect your body. Use your common sense when practicing and become aware of how your body feels as it performs the stretches.

Zen Yoga practice is not a competition. It is an internal self-discipline. It makes no difference what someone else is able to do. The photographs in this section are representations of the way the stretch is supposed to look. However, do not try to force yourself into a position your body is not ready for. Simply try to stretch to your own ability. Every body is different. Learn what your own body can and cannot do.

The following exercises are a sample of the infinite possibilities that exist within the practice of Zen Yoga. They will assist you in teaching yourself to move, stretch, and breathe in ways that make you feel good. They are a good sequence for beginners to start out with after warm-up. You are encouraged to expand these after you get the hang of them. Keep an open mind. Use the ones that work for you. Drop the ones you don't like. Invent new ones that feel right for you. Add more repetitions or lengthen the time of stretch if you find it beneficial. Most important, enjoy. The whole idea is to open new spaces and then breathe into those spaces. Direct the breath with your mind. If you can't feel it, imagine it. Your mind will lead the energy there.

Stretching

STARBURST

Lying flat on your back, stretch your arms and legs out as if being pulled in all directions at the same time. Imagine you are waking up for the first time in your life, and expand so that you stretch out every muscle in your body, like a starburst. Feel the stretch from the center of your being to the outer reaches of the universe. Reach out, stretch out, and breathe deeply, allowing the breath to fill the open spaces in your body. Once you have reached your extension, drop the tension and let your body become a lead weight, sinking into the ground. Focus on your breath as it enters and leaves your body.

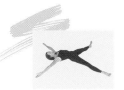

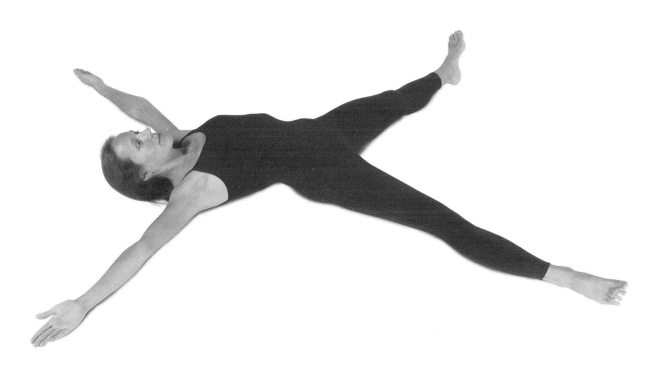

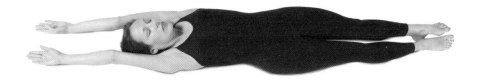

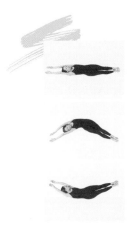

CRESCENT MOON

Lying flat on your back with your arms on the ground above your head, lengthen and extend through your spine while you stretch your arms and legs. "Walk" your legs together to one side and then move your arms together to the same side so that your body arcs into the shape of a crescent moon. Try to keep your shoulders and hips flat on the ground. One side of your body is now contracted while the other is open. Extend and lengthen from your fingertips to your toes, breathe into the open side of your body and feel the breath filling you. Replicate on the other side.

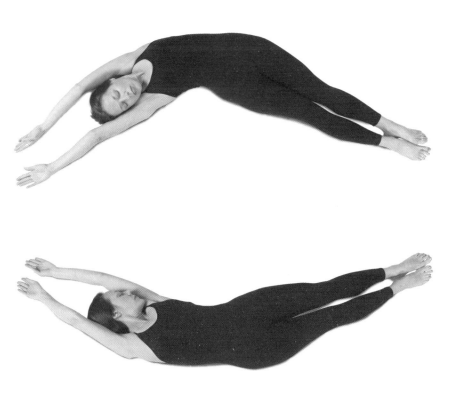

TWIST

Lying flat on your back with your arms extended out to the side, bend your knees and bring them up toward your chest. Keeping your knees together, gently lower them to the floor on your right, beneath the right elbow. Turn your head to the left. Place your right hand on top of your left knee in order to apply a little pressure to the stretch. Breathe into the abdomen. Since the body is twisted, it may feel a little constricted. Try to push the breath back toward the spine. This brings the energy directly to the area being stretched. Repeat on the other side. When you finish both sides, bring your knees back up to your chest and clasp them with your hands. Gently rock from side to side massaging the spine. Release the legs and relax.

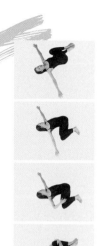

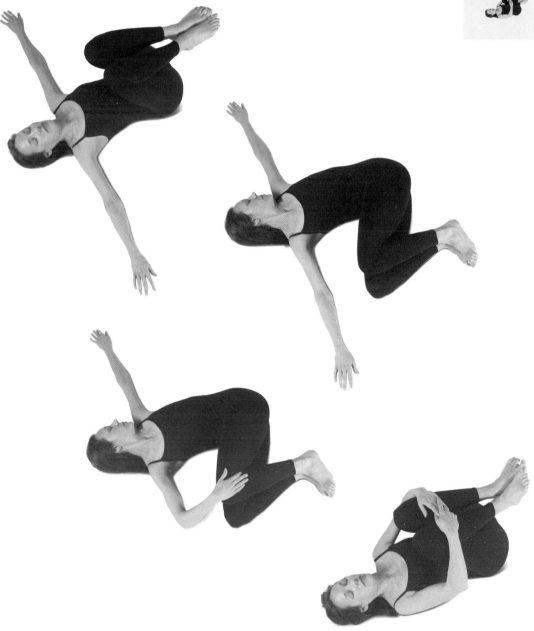

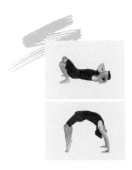

WHEEL

The Wheel is an advanced pose that requires arm and back strength. Please take care. Lying on your back, bend your knees keeping your feet on the floor near the buttocks. Bring your hands up to the side of your head and place your palms on the floor, fingertips near your shoulders, pointing toward your feet. Breathe in deeply and, as you exhale, press down with your arms and legs while raising your torso toward the sky. Extend through your knees and elbows. Relax your neck. Continue to breathe. In this position your breathing can be a little restricted, but try to keep it strong and continuous.

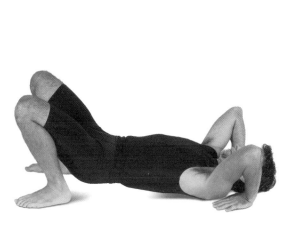

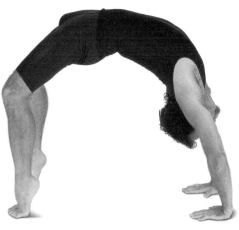

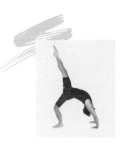

■ Extended Wheel
If you have the strength, bring one foot closer to center and raise the other foot up over your body. Point the toes and extend the leg. Continue breathing strongly and smoothly.

CAT ARCH

From a kneeling position, with arms forward and palms flat on the floor, come up onto your fingertips. Sink your weight back slightly and curl your chin into the chest, forming a curve in the back that extends down to the tail bone. Curl the hips forward and draw your navel up. Breathe and feel the expansion of the area of your back along the curve of the spine. Hold the position for at least three breaths.

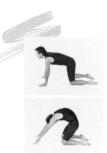

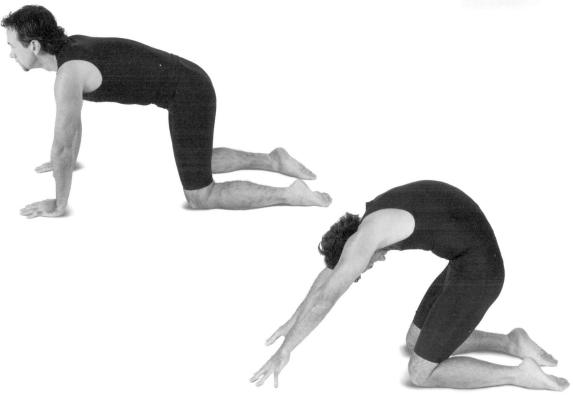

EARTH PRAYER

From a kneeling position, sink back on your heels so you are resting on the backs of your legs. With your arms outstretched, pull the shoulders away from the torso. Bow the head down between the arms. Feel the compression of your diaphragm against the tops of your thighs as you breathe. Hold the position for at least three breaths.

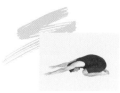

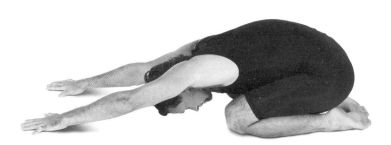

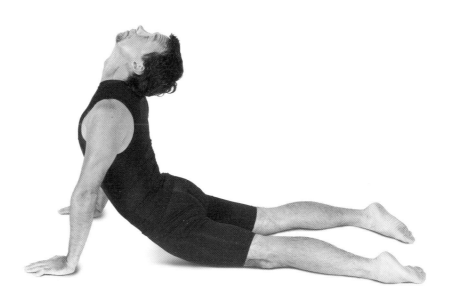

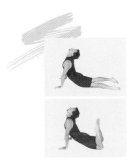

COBRA ARCH

Lying on your front with your palms down under your shoulders, press into the floor with your hands and raise your head and chest. Push your hips and legs into the floor and feel as if your chest is rising out of your lower body. Drop your head back. Breathe as deeply as you can while feeling your belly compress against the floor. If you are able, bend at the knees and raise both feet toward the sky. Point the toes. Hold for three breaths.

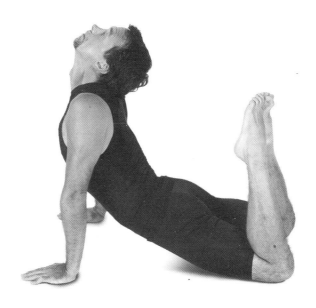

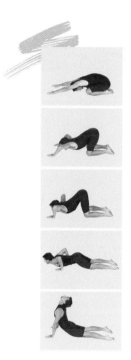

COBRA GLIDE

Starting from the Earth Prayer position, breathe in. Keeping your head and chest low to the ground, breathe out as you glide through between your arms until your body is extended along the floor. Push into the palms of your hands and straighten your arms as you rise up into the Cobra Arch. Breathe in again as you raise your chin and look up. Breathe out. Retrace the path back to the Earth Prayer position.

When doing this exercise, use your whole body. Legs, hips, arms, and back all work together, moving smoothly and continuously. Don't be discouraged if you don't have the strength to do it perfectly the first time, do the best you can. With regular practice you will soon be able to feel your whole body moving in a coordinated effort.

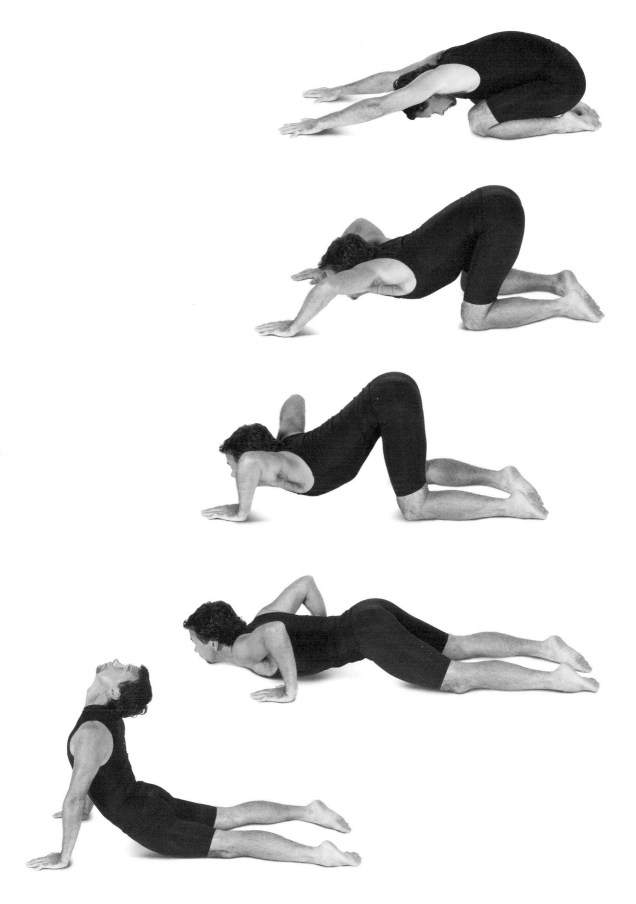

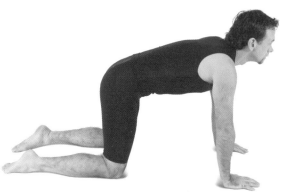

KNEELING KICK

From a kneeling position, raise your right leg and extend it up and back. Raise your head, look forward, and breathe in. Breathe out as you bring your extended leg forward toward the chest. Drop your head down, trying to touch your forehead to your knee. Next, inhale as you extend your leg back out and raise your head. Exhale again as you contract your knee to your forehead. Repeat the Kneeling Kick five times and then replicate with the other leg.

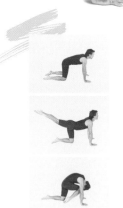

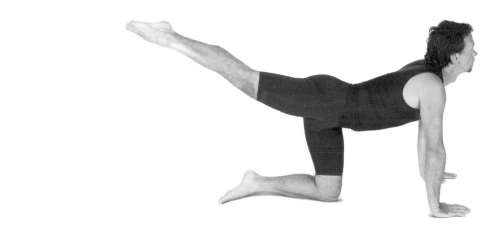

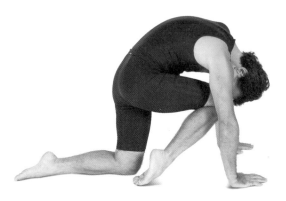

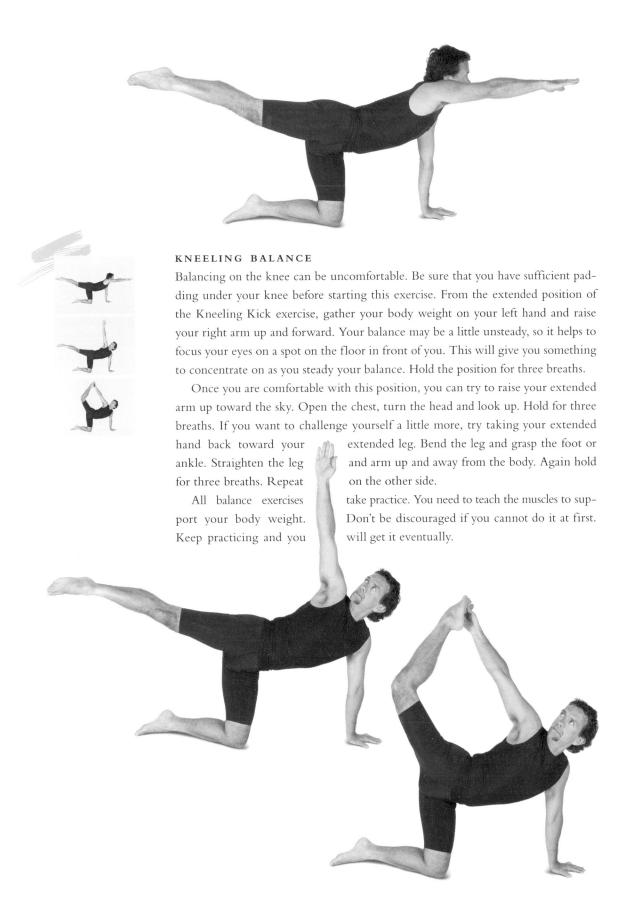

KNEELING BALANCE

Balancing on the knee can be uncomfortable. Be sure that you have sufficient padding under your knee before starting this exercise. From the extended position of the Kneeling Kick exercise, gather your body weight on your left hand and raise your right arm up and forward. Your balance may be a little unsteady, so it helps to focus your eyes on a spot on the floor in front of you. This will give you something to concentrate on as you steady your balance. Hold the position for three breaths.

Once you are comfortable with this position, you can try to raise your extended arm up toward the sky. Open the chest, turn the head and look up. Hold for three breaths. If you want to challenge yourself a little more, try taking your extended hand back toward your extended leg. Bend the leg and grasp the foot or ankle. Straighten the leg and arm up and away from the body. Again hold for three breaths. Repeat on the other side.

All balance exercises take practice. You need to teach the muscles to support your body weight. Don't be discouraged if you cannot do it at first. Keep practicing and you will get it eventually.

CAMEL ARCH

Sit on your heels and place your hands on your heels or upturned feet. Gradually raise your weight up off your legs and push your pelvis forward. Keeping your hands on your heels, open your chest and release your neck muscles to let your head arc back. Try to hold the position for three breaths as you lengthen through your arms.

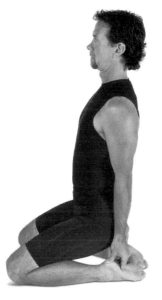

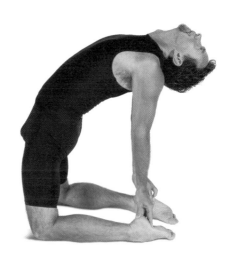

■ Extended Camel

This is an advanced exercise that requires a lot of strength in the back; approach it with caution. From the Camel Arch tighten the muscles in your lower back to support your weight and lift the arms up and back, away from the body. Lean back, extend your arms and breathe.

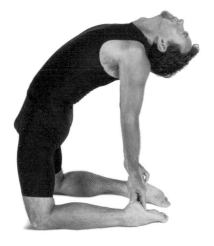

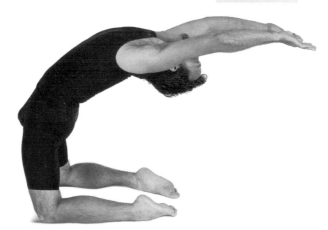

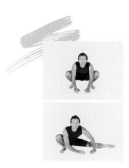

■ Dragon Stretch

From a squatting position, extend one leg out to the side. Keeping your arms in front of you to support your body weight, sink your rear end down and lengthen through the hamstring of the extended leg. Keep both hands in front of you to take some of the weight. Flex your ankles. It is not necessary to put the heel of your supporting leg on the floor. Raise your chin. Breathe and relax into the stretch for at least three breaths. Shift to the other side, using your hands to support your weight.

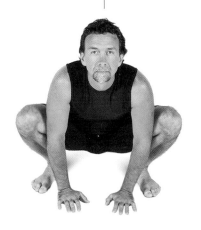

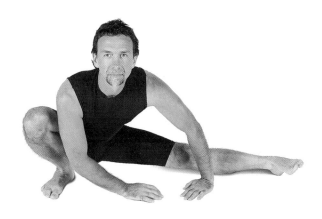

■ Dragon Lunge

From the Dragon Stretch position rotate your hips out over your bent knee, rolling your extended leg over and pointing your toes. Place your hands on either side of your front foot and place your upper body along your front thigh. Lengthen your back leg and stretch through the hip joint. Lift your back knee off the ground if that feels more comfortable. Hold the position for three breaths.

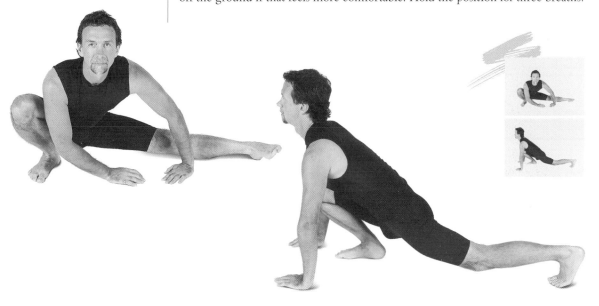

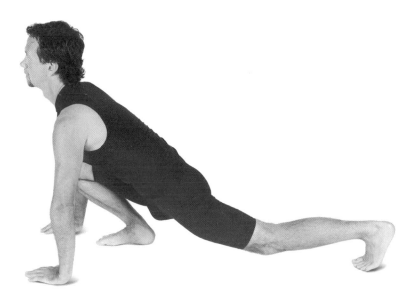

■ Drop Hip

From the Dragon Lunge position drop the hip of your extended leg toward the floor, twist your hips and turn your head to look back over your shoulder. Try to have the whole leg from hip to ankle touching the floor. Breathe into the stretched hip and hold for three breaths.

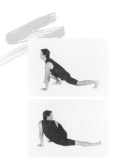

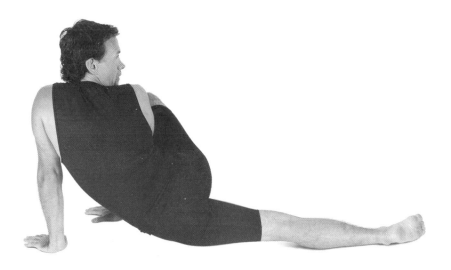

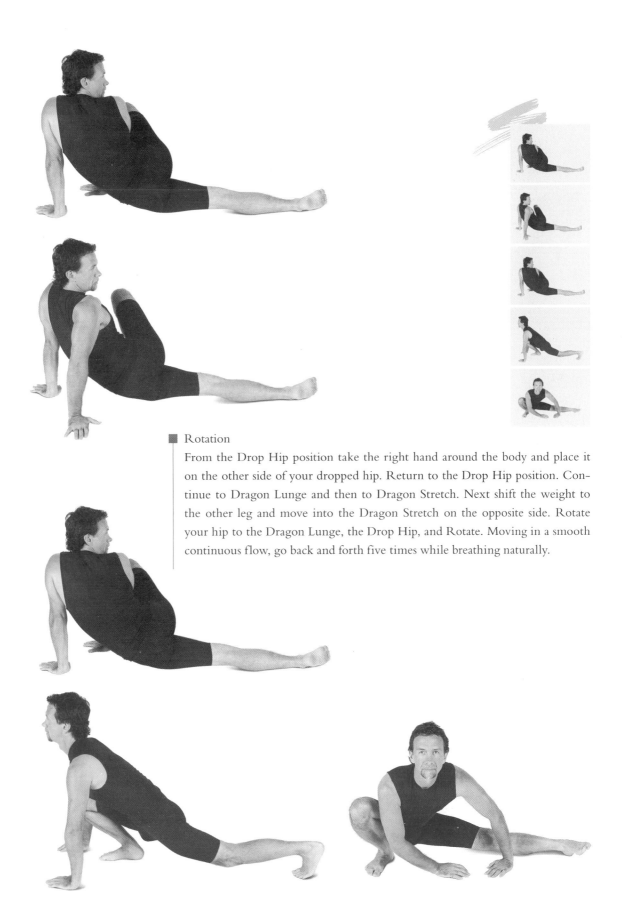

Rotation

From the Drop Hip position take the right hand around the body and place it on the other side of your dropped hip. Return to the Drop Hip position. Continue to Dragon Lunge and then to Dragon Stretch. Next shift the weight to the other leg and move into the Dragon Stretch on the opposite side. Rotate your hip to the Dragon Lunge, the Drop Hip, and Rotate. Moving in a smooth continuous flow, go back and forth five times while breathing naturally.

■ Cobra Pigeon

From the Dragon Lunge position push the knee out toward the floor and reposition the foot so that the lower leg is on the floor in front of you. Your heel should be just near your navel. Press your palms into the floor and raise your head and chest up and back. Push your hips forward and feel as if your chest is rising out of your lower body. Drop your head back. Hold the position for three breaths.

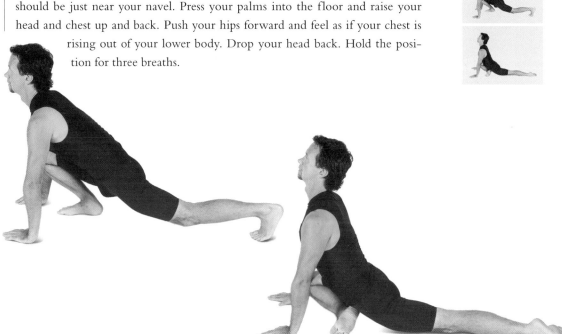

■ Extended Pigeon

From the Cobra Pigeon position, extend your arms out in front of you and lay the upper body down over the bent front leg. Extend the arms forward, stretching from the armpits. Allow the heel of your foot to press into your abdomen and focus your breathing there. Hold for three breaths.

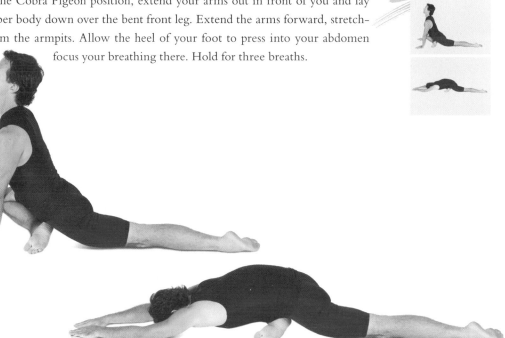

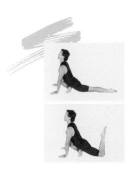

■ Tail Up

From the Cobra Pigeon position, bend the back knee and raise the foot to the sky. Point the toes. Breathe deeply for three breaths.

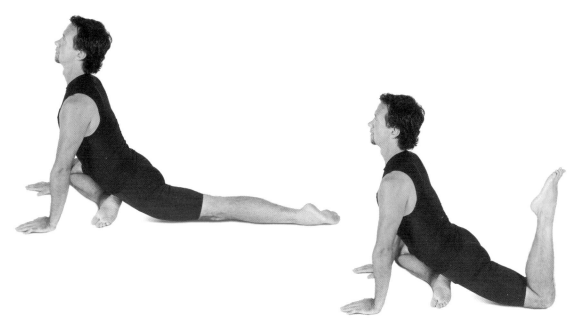

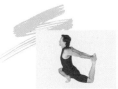

■ Clasp Tail

From the Tail Up position, reach back with one hand and grasp your raised foot. Once you get your balance, see if you can also reach back with the other hand to grasp that foot. Continue to hold the position for three breaths.

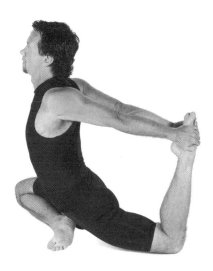

■ Straight Split

From a standing position spread the legs out away from each other. Open the legs as far apart as you can. When you reach your maximum extension reach down to the floor and gently ease yourself to a sitting position maintaining the open leg position. Once you are seated, straighten the back and sit up. Breathe and let yourself relax into the stretch. Hold the position for at least three breaths, and then gradually increase the number once you are comfortable with the position.

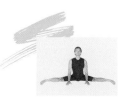

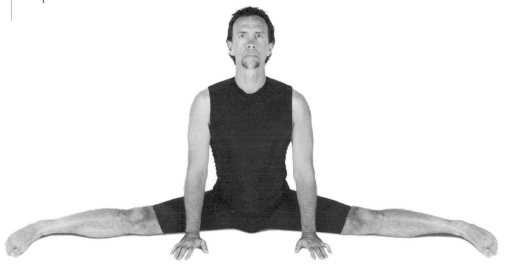

■ Toes Up

From the Straight Split position, point your toes up to the sky. Next point your toes out away from your legs. Alternate between these two positions and feel the muscles in your legs adjusting with each move. Repeat five times.

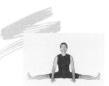

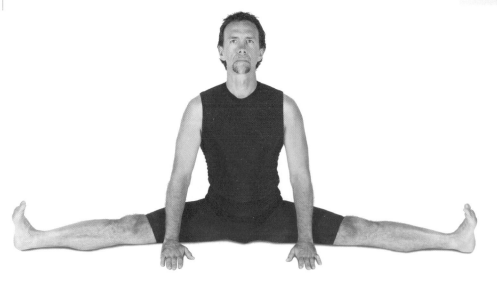

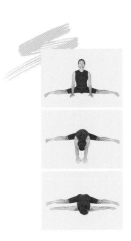

Forward

From the Straight Split position, point your toes forward, rotating the whole leg from the hip joint. Bring your arms forward and slowly walk your upper body down toward the front. Stop at whatever point is your maximum stretch. Breathe in, and as you exhale allow the muscles of your legs to relax. Once you have taken a couple of breaths you should be able to extend forward a little deeper. If you can come forward to the floor, try to extend your arms out to the side and rest your body weight on your chest. Hold that position for at least three breaths.

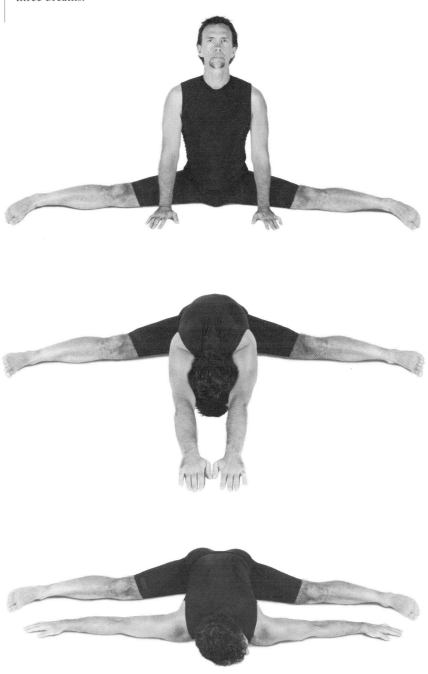

■ Side Bend Split

From the Toes Up position, reach out to one side toward the toes. If you cannot reach your toes, your ankle or shin is fine. Drop your elbow to your knee and raise your other hand up over your head. Lengthen your upper body and lay it down along the length of your leg, dropping your raised hand toward the toes as well. Again, breathing slowly will allow you to relax deeper into the stretch. Repeat to the other side.

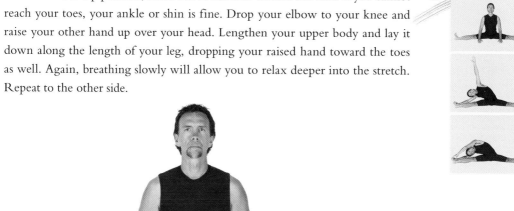

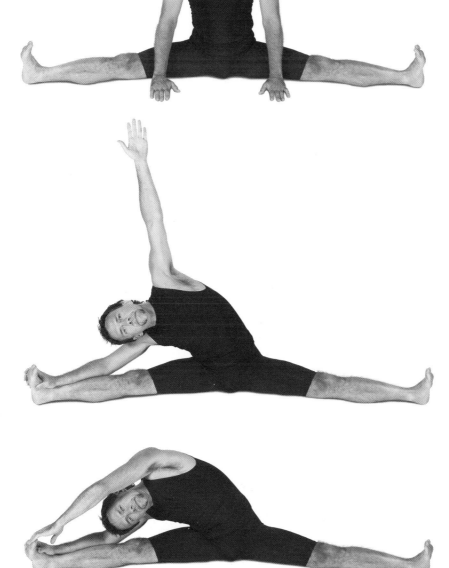

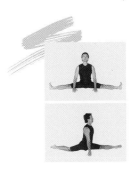

FRONT SPLIT

From a straight split position, place one hand in front between your legs and the other hand behind you. Turn toward the side as you rotate the hips into the split. This is a difficult stretch and you will need to support your weight on your arms as you rotate your hips. Turn your back leg so the knee is down on the floor and point your back toes. Hold the position for a few moments and try to maintain slow relaxed breathing while concentrating on the stretch. If this is easy you can try to bend your head down toward your front leg. Repeat the stretch facing the other way.

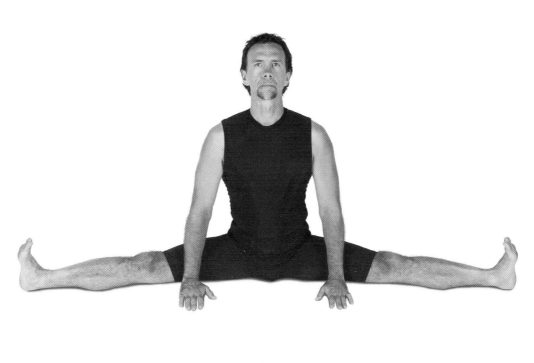

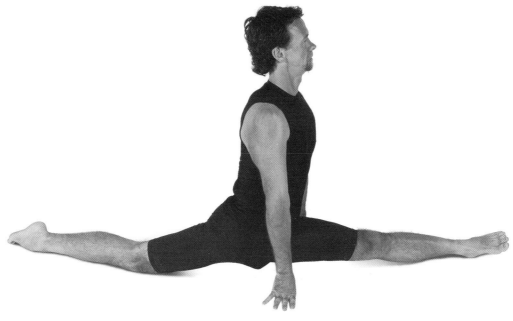

JUXTAPOSE

Sit on the floor with the knees bent and your feet on the floor pointing away at 45 degree angles. Drop one knee inwards to the ground while leaving the other leg stationary. Hold the position for three breaths. Repeat on the other side.

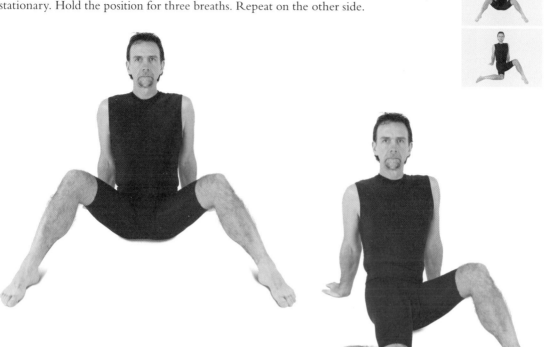

FORWARD BEND

From a sitting position, legs straight out in front of you, raise your arms above your head and bend forward so that your upper body is extended above the lower body. Drop your head toward your knees. Reach to your toes. If this is too difficult, grab the ankles or anywhere else along your legs that is comfortable. Breathe and relax into the stretch. Hold for at least three breaths.

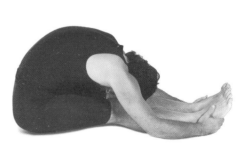

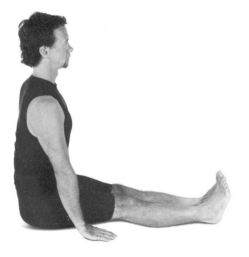

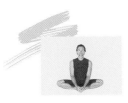

BUTTERFLY

Sit on the floor and pull both feet into the body. Place the bottoms of the feet together and pull them in toward the body. Keep your back straight and breathe as your legs relax into the stretch. You can gently raise and lower your knees for a little more stretch in the groin area. Breathing should be relaxed and natural.

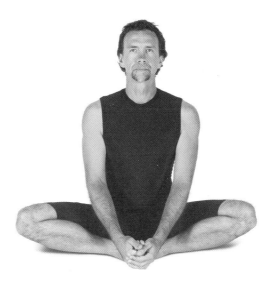

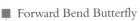

■ Forward Bend Butterfly

From the Butterfly position, pull your feet as close into the body as possible. Lengthen your back and bend forward. Try to bring your head down to touch your feet. Focus on breathing deeper and hold the position for at least three breaths.

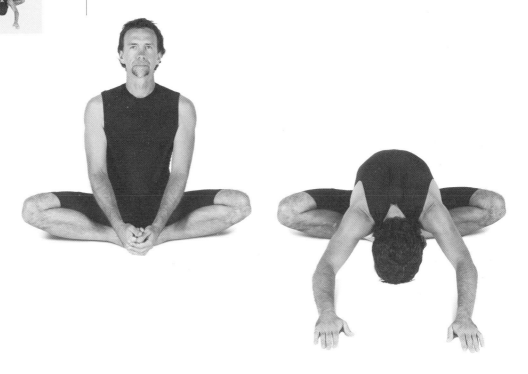

FROG

Kneel on the floor. Walk your hands forward as you push your knees apart. Arch your back slightly and bring your feet together behind you. Drop you hips and pelvis down toward the floor as you open you knees. Hold and breathe for three full breaths.

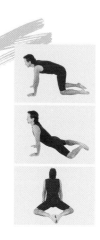

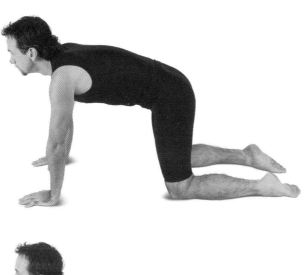

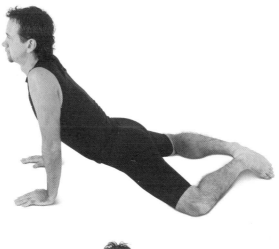

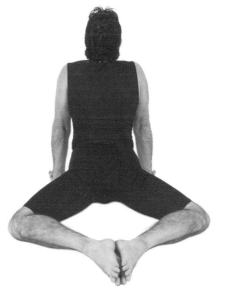

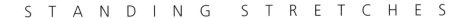

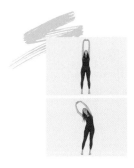

UPWARD EXTENSION

From a normal standing position, interlock the fingers and raise your arms above your head. Reach straight and tall, stretching your arms up and out from the shoulders. Lengthen the torso and extend up and out of your hips. Reach high as you raise your chin and look up. Lightly bend from side to side. Remember to breathe naturally and continuously.

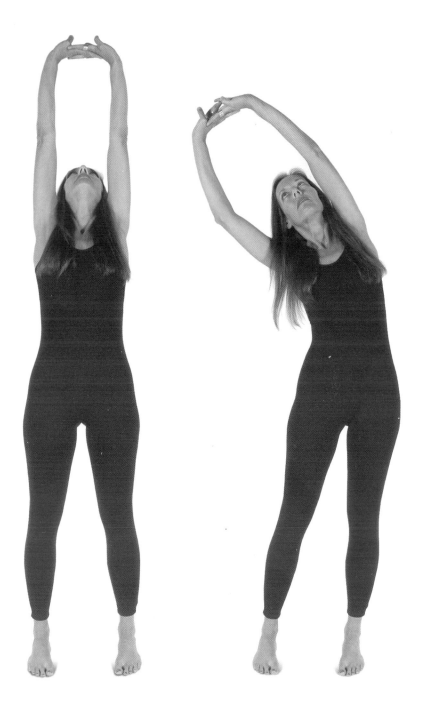

■ Elephant Twist

From a standing position, bend forward at the waist. Imagine your arms are elephant trunks and gently sway them back and forth around your legs. There should be no strength or tension in your dangling arms: let it go. Feel the stretch in the backs of your legs as well as your lower back area. Breathe and let go. Continue swaying for three breaths.

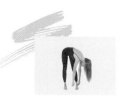

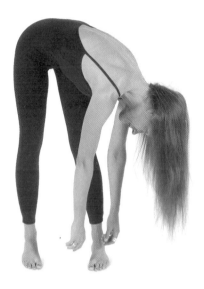

■ Tail Wag

In the Forward Bend position, touch your fingertips to the floor. Unlock your knees and bend them if necessary to enable you to touch the floor. Gently sway your hips from side to side, stretching the lower back and kidney area. Continue the motion for at least three breaths.

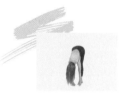

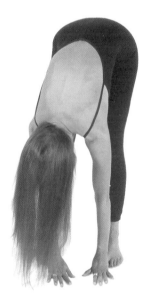

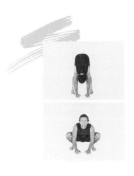

ZEN SQUAT

From a Forward Bend position, bend at the knees and squat down over your feet using your hands for balance to support your weight. Feel the stretch in your lower back, hips, knees, and ankles. If you are able, press your heels onto the floor. Raise your chin and look ahead. Breathe in a natural and relaxed manner.

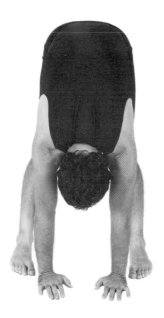

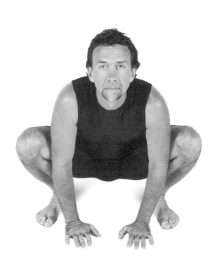

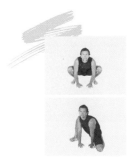

■ Knee Down

From the Zen Squat position, bend one knee forward to touch the ground in front of you. Push the other knee out and back, opening the hip and stretching the legs and ankles. Repeat using the other leg. Alternate five times while breathing.

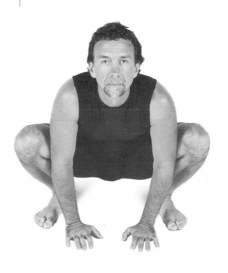

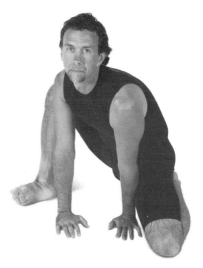

■ Raise Hips

From the Zen Squat position, inhale and raise your tailbone to the sky. Exhale and return to the Zen Squat position. Repeat five times, being sure to completely inhale as you rise up and completely exhale as you return to the squat position.

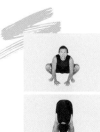

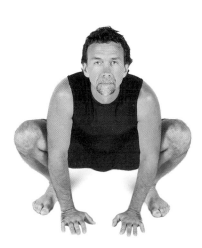

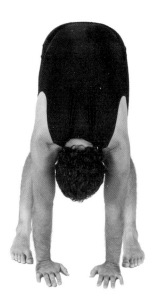

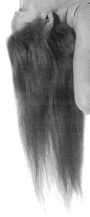

BACKWARD BEND

From a standing position place both hands at the lower back with the palms inward. Rise up tall out of the hips and bend backwards. Raise your chin to the sky. Breathing can be a little difficult in this position, but be sure to continue pushing the breath down to the abdomen.

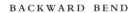

SIDE BEND

From a standing position, raise one hand straight above the head. Slowly slide the other hand down the leg toward the knee. Bend at the waist, supporting your weight with the lower arm. Feel as if you are closing one side of your body and opening the other. Breathe into the open side as you stretch from your fingertips along the arc of your body. Hold for three breaths and then repeat on the other side.

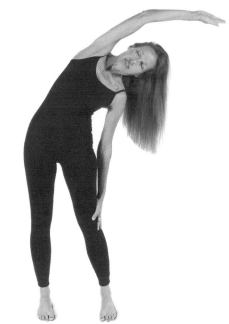

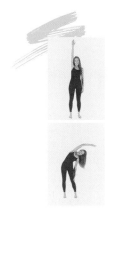

■ Rotate In

From the Side Bend stretched position, turn your upper shoulder inward and drop your raised arm toward your ankle. Bring your head down to the side of your knee. Unlock the muscles of the back and ribs as you breathe. Hold for at least three breaths and then repeat on the other side.

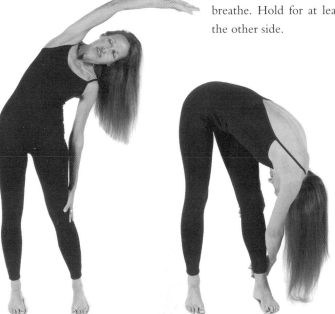

OPEN & CLAP

Standing straight, raise both arms in front and put the palms together. Leave the right hand in that position as you rotate to the left and open your left arm, taking it back behind you. Turn your hips and shoulders, opening your chest. Swing the arm back to the front and clap the hands together. Rotate to the other side taking the right hand back. Repeat five times.

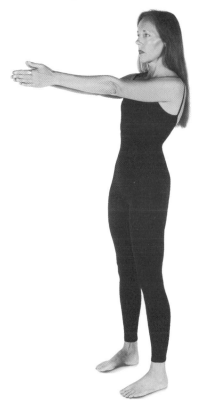

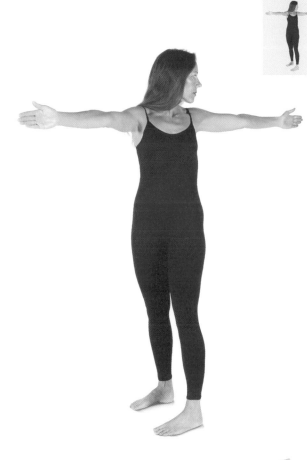

ZEN DOG

From a kneeling position on all fours, tuck your toes under and straighten your legs. Keep your head down between your outstretched arms as your hips rise up. Push your heels back and lengthen your back by stretching your chest down toward the floor. Feel the stretch along your legs, back, and arms. Hold for three breaths.

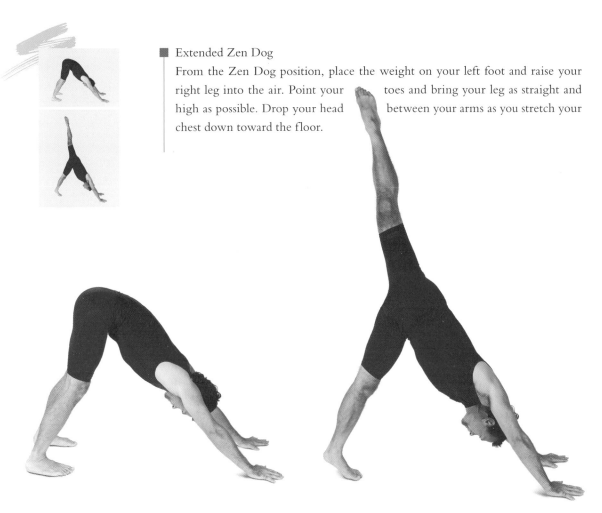

■ Extended Zen Dog

From the Zen Dog position, place the weight on your left foot and raise your right leg into the air. Point your toes and bring your leg as straight and high as possible. Drop your head between your arms as you stretch your chest down toward the floor.

CHIN TO TOE

From the Forward Bend position, shift one foot forward slightly. Flex the ankle and pull the toes up toward your chin. Reach out with your hands and grasp the foot of that leg. Lengthen your body along that leg. Grasping your foot, begin to stretch down toward it, drawing your head toward your toes. The goal of this exercise is to touch your chin to your big toe while keeping the leg straight. If anyone is actually able to accomplish this incredibly difficult stretch, please send a photo to my website and I will post it on a special page.

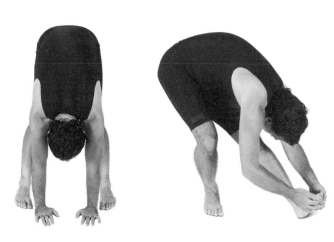

I N V E R S I O N S

Inversions are a wonderful method for helping to get Zen energy to flow through the body more effectively. Inversions turn things upside down and use the natural pull of gravity to assist in changing and strengthening the blood flow through the body. Inversions are advanced exercises and are not recommended until you have reached the proper level of fitness and body awareness. Because of the physical requirements, inversions should be approached cautiously. While very beneficial for the body, inversions have inherent dangers and should be done with proper care and attention. Anyone with doubts about the suitability of the exercises should consult a doctor before attempting them.

SHOULDER STAND SERIES

Lie on your back with your legs extended. Bend your legs and bring the knees up above your chest, using your hands to prop up your back. Allow the weight of your body to be supported by your shoulders, elbows, and neck. Straighten your legs. Tuck your chin into your chest. Breathe while you alternate between pointing your toes and flexing your ankles.

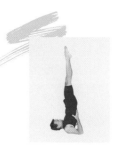

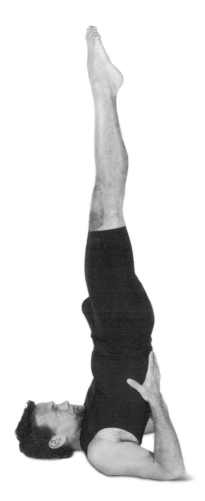

Plow

From the Shoulder Stand position take both legs over your head toward the floor. Flex your ankles and try to bring your feet to the floor. Drop your arms back to the floor behind you. Feel the stretch through your legs and back. Concentrate on breathing deeply even though you will feel a bit constricted. Hold for three breaths.

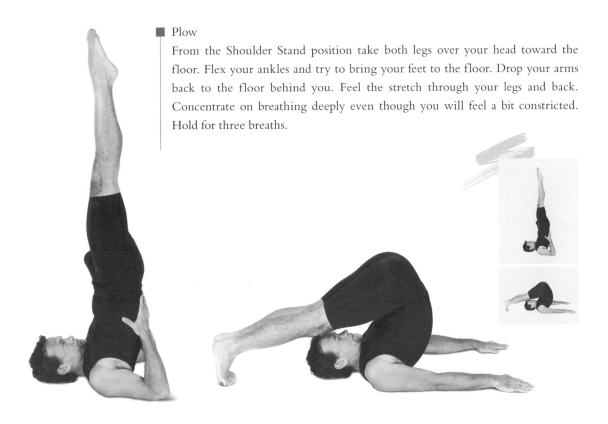

Extended Plow

From the Plow position, raise one leg up into the air above the body and point your toes. Lengthen and extend your stretched leg. Hold for three breaths, then switch legs.

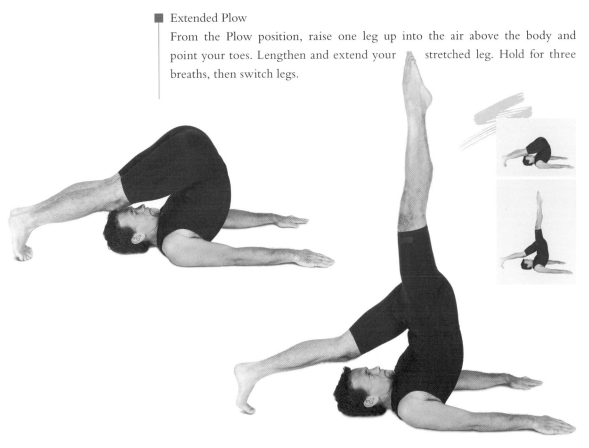

■ Jackknife

The Jackknife position is the same as the Plow position, except that here you bring your arms up and extend them along the floor under your legs. Try to reach your feet with your hands while focused on your breathing. You should feel the stretch in your upper back, arms, and legs. Hold for three breaths.

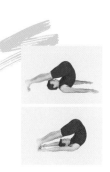

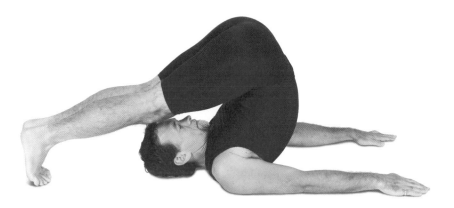

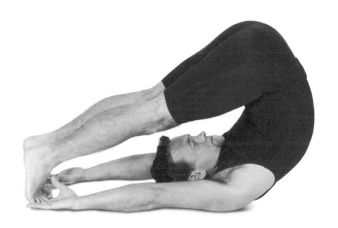

HEADSTAND

Since much of the weight of the body is supported by the head, it is advisable to use a pillow or folded blanket during headstand practice. It may also be helpful to have a fitness instructor or friend spot you by holding your legs up to keep them steady. Headstands involve a rush of blood to the head and pressure on the brain and eyes. People with high blood pressure, the elderly, and overweight people should not attempt these exercises. Always make sure you have plenty of space around you in case you lose your balance.

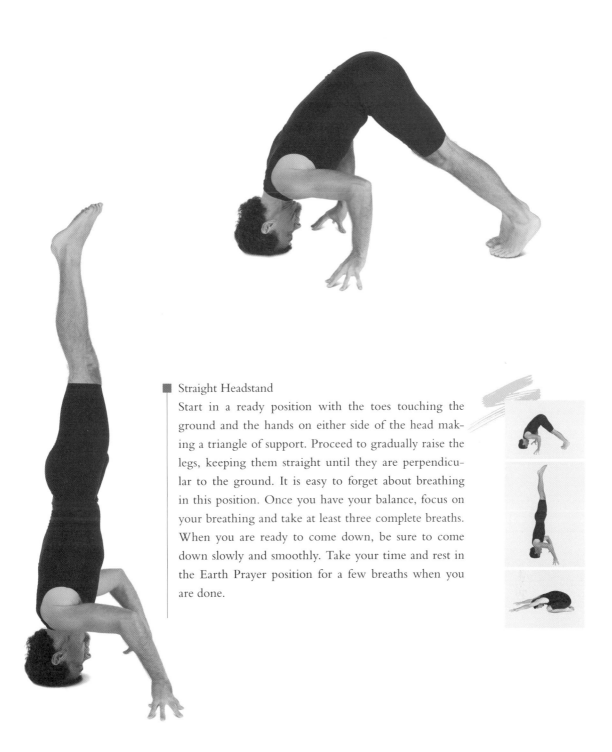

Straight Headstand

Start in a ready position with the toes touching the ground and the hands on either side of the head making a triangle of support. Proceed to gradually raise the legs, keeping them straight until they are perpendicular to the ground. It is easy to forget about breathing in this position. Once you have your balance, focus on your breathing and take at least three complete breaths. When you are ready to come down, be sure to come down slowly and smoothly. Take your time and rest in the Earth Prayer position for a few breaths when you are done.

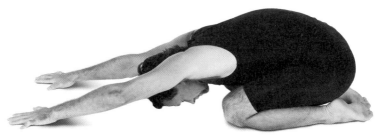

■ Split Headstand

From the Straight Headstand position open your legs and extend them out and down. Take care to move them simultaneously so that you can maintain your balance. Once you are in position, focus on your breathing and hold for three breaths.

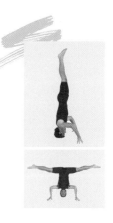

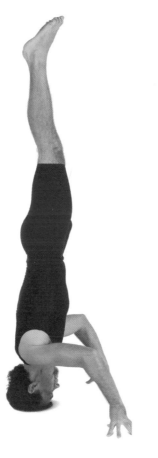

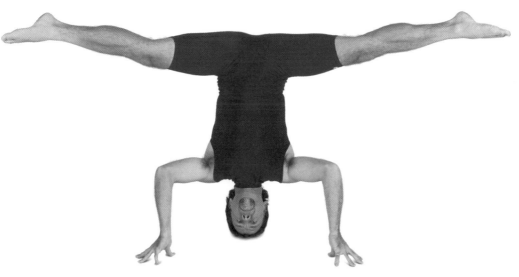

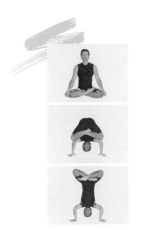

Lotus Headstand

This is an advanced headstand position and it is recommended that you practice the Straight Headstand before attempting this. From a Lotus Sitting position, lean forward and place your head on the ground. Using your abdominal muscles raise your knees up to rest on your elbows. When you are ready, raise the knees up to the sky maintaining your legs in Lotus position. Return to your breathing and hold the position for three breaths.

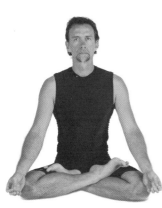

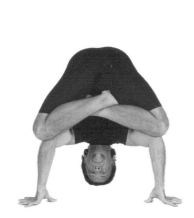

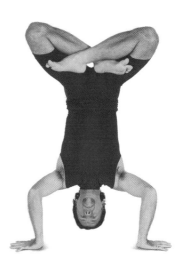

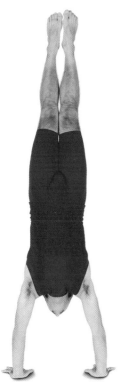

HANDSTAND

The Handstand can be difficult to maintain because of the arm strength required to support the weight of the body. It is very helpful to practice against a wall for support until you are comfortable and strong enough to support your full weight. Bend forward and, with arms straight, place your hands on the ground. Swing your legs up over your head. You may need to make adjustments by walking on your hands until you get your balance. Handstands take a lot of patience and practice. Don't be discouraged. It can take more than a year of regular practice before you are able to hold the position for more than a few seconds.

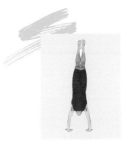

SCORPION

Scorpion is another advanced pose that takes time, patience, and strength to execute properly. It can take quite a while for your arms and shoulders to acquire the strength to hold your body weight.

◼ Straight Scorpion
Kneel on the floor with your hands and elbows on the ground in front of you. Raise the legs as if you were going to do a handstand but support yourself on your elbows and forearms. Support your weight evenly on your forearms and raise both legs up straight. Find your balance and breathe. Hold the position for three breaths if possible.

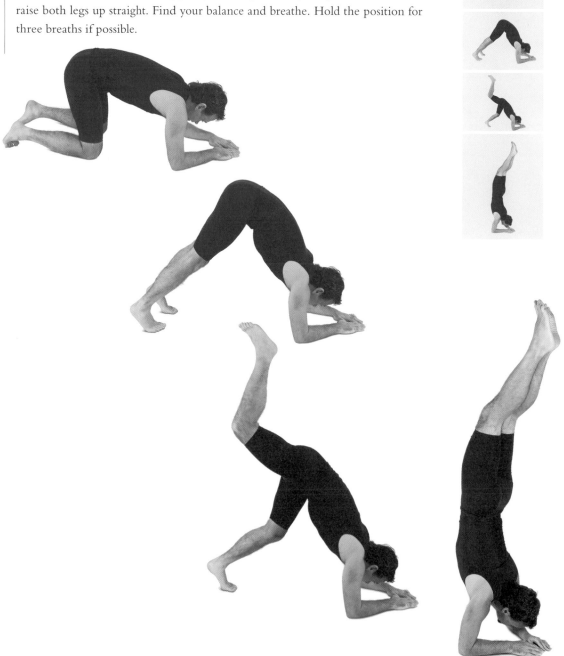

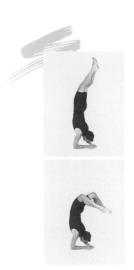

■ Scorpion Tail

From the Straight Scorpion position, bend your legs at the knees and let your feet hang forward, toward the back of your head. Breathe as you work to maintain your balance.

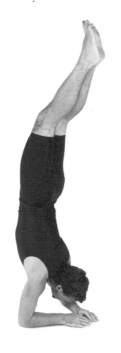

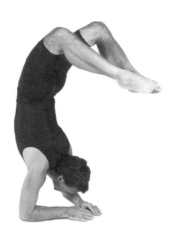

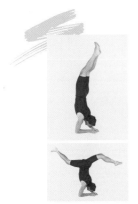

■ Scorpion Split

From the Straight Scorpion position, extend one leg forward and the other back into a split position. Take care to maintain your balance as you adjust your weight. Hold the position for three breaths, then switch legs.

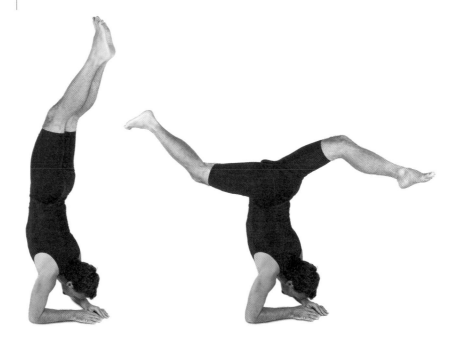

BASIC

Basic balance exercises are usually accessible to anyone. However they can be challenging if you have not done any balancing before. The secret to balance is in understanding that it is not the large muscles of the body that are important when practicing balance. Instead, it is the subtle, minor, supporting muscles of your legs that make the corrections and adjustments in order maintain balance. In order to strengthen them it is helpful to practice these Zen Yoga Balance positions. Work into the positions slowly, however, allowing your body to become used to the challenge.

■ Tree

Stand with your feet together and straighten your arms above your head. Clasp your palms together. Shift the weight to the left leg and slowly raise the heel of the right foot off the floor. Bring it over to the left leg and place it behind the left calf. Slowly raise the right leg until your right foot is resting behind your left knee. Raise your chin and look up at your hands as you breathe. You should feel yourself lengthening and extending from your hips upwards. Pull your elbows close together and reach up. Replicate on other side.

■ Elbow over Knee

Stand with your feet shoulder-width apart. Extend your right arm forward and bend it at the elbow ninety degrees so that the hand is pointing up. Raise your right leg off the floor and, pointing the knee forward, continue to lift it until it is waist height or higher. Align the elbow over the knee as you maintain your balance. Focus on your breathing and hold for three breaths. Replicate on the other side.

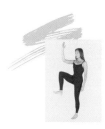

MODERATE STANCES

These Moderate stances are more challenging. They incorporate the arms into the balance and, consequently, are more stressful on a variety of muscles. Concentration is important. It will still your mind and aid in maintaining your balance. Focusing your gaze on a fixed point, either on the floor or in your line of vision, sometimes helps control balance.

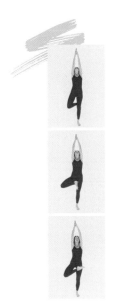

■ Advanced Tree

From the Basic Tree position, bring the leg up higher so that the bottom of the foot is pressed against the inside of the upper thigh of the supporting leg. Another variation of this is to place the foot on top of the thigh. Reach the arms high above your head with the palms together; lengthen up and out of the hips. Stretch high and raise your chin to the sky. Hold the position for three breaths and then replicate on the other side.

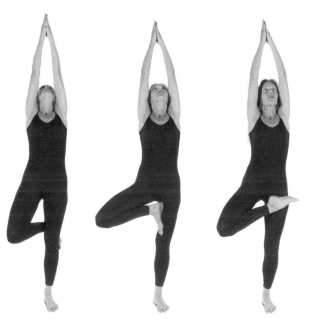

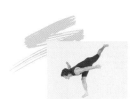

■ Airplane

Stand on one leg and stretch the other one out behind you in the air. Stretch both arms out away from the body. Tilt the whole body forward allowing the back foot to rise up. Bend the supporting knee slightly. Maintain this position for three breaths, then lower your outstretched leg and repeat for the other one.

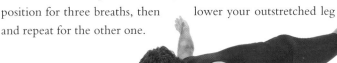

DIFFICULT

Difficult balance positions are not for everyone. They place considerable strain on the muscles and joints. Do not attempt them unless you are physically fit and flexible enough to handle the added strain.

■ Extend Front

Raise your right knee up and grab your toes with your right hand. Slowly extend your leg forward and out as you straighten your arm, lengthening through your knee and armpit. Bend your supporting leg and let your weight sink down. Hold for three breaths and then repeat with the other leg.

■ Extend Side

Bring the right leg up and point the knee out to the side. Grab the outside of the foot with your right hand. Slowly extend your leg out to the side and up as you lengthen your arm. Bend your supporting leg and sink your weight down. Hold for three breaths and then repeat with the other leg.

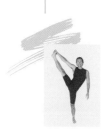

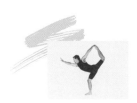

■ Extend Back

Bring your left foot up behind you
and point the knee to the ground.
Grab the top of the foot with your left hand.
Extend your right hand forward and slowly raise
your leg up and back. Bend your supporting knee
and tilt your upper body forward. Raise the leg
and knee higher, extending through the hip. Hold
for three breaths and then repeat with the other
leg.

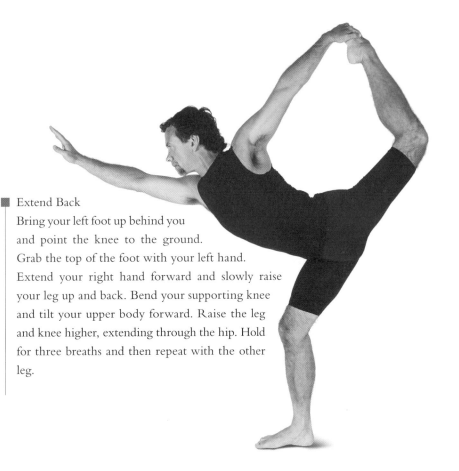

CHAPTER

6

Relaxation Exercises

You have powers you never dreamed of,
You can do things you never thought you could do,
There are no limitations...
Except the limitations of your own mind.

—A. H.

Beginning

Relaxing exercises are the heart and soul of building a strong energy flow. You can breathe and stretch all you like, but if your mind is running a hundred miles per minute and you are stressed or anxious, you will never be able to reach the state of being for which you have the potential. Physical tension is a substantial barrier. Until you can pierce this barrier, you will not be able to affect the inner layers of yourself. Focusing your mind and learning to deal with stress can be difficult if not impossible until you have let go of your tensions and reduced the pain and discomfort of your physical body.

T E N S I O N   R E L E A S E

Tension Release is about teaching the body to surrender. It is the unclenching and unwinding of the musculature as you learn to let go. The simplest and quickest method for releasing tension within the body involves contrasting tension with relaxation. If we bear in mind the basic idea of yin and yang, we can readily grasp this concept. It calls for forcing the body to experience the extremes of tension so that when balanced by an equally full experience of relaxation, the latter becomes much more pronounced, identifiable, and deeper.

SQUEEZE

Begin by lying flat on your back, legs straight and your feet flopped apart. Close your eyes and take a few natural breaths as your body settles down. When you are ready, begin deep Basic Abdominal Breathing (page 44); inhale through your nose, expand your lungs, push out, and fill up completely. Stop. Hold in your breath. As you do so curl your toes, and squeeze your feet as tightly as possible. Hold the squeeze for a moment and then release it as you exhale through the nose.

Begin again. Fill your lungs and hold. This time, once you curl your toes and squeeze your feet, squeeze your calf muscles, thigh muscles, and buttocks. Tense all of your muscles from the hips down, so that your whole lower body is tight and rigid. Hold the squeeze for a moment and then release it as you exhale. Let go of all the muscles. Allow them to uncoil and unwind.

Next, as you breathe in, imagine you are filling up the lowest areas of your body and allowing the breath to penetrate deep into your being. Visualize the oxygen-rich blood coursing through the clear passages into your legs.

When you are ready, begin again. Fill your lungs and hold. This time—once you have curled your toes and squeezed your feet, calves, thighs, and buttocks— begin to tighten the muscles of the stomach. Squeeze the ribcage, chest, and muscles under your armpits. Hold the squeeze for a moment and then release it as you exhale. Let go of all the muscles. Allow them to completely release and let go. Breathe and rest as you allow your body to be filled with energy. Take note of any new or different feelings within your body.

Once again breathe in and fill up. Hold in your breath and curl your toes, squeeze your feet, calves, thighs and buttocks, stomach, ribs, chest, and underarms. Next make tight fists with your hands. Tighten your elbows, shoulders, and neck muscles. Squeeze your eyes tight shut, grit your teeth, and squeeze your whole body for just a moment. Then release it as you breathe out a long, slow exhalation. Let go of all the muscles. Feel yourself sinking down into the ground as all of the tension is drained out of you.

Continue to take long, deep breaths and feel the energy flowing through your body.

Your body learns through active participation. In this exercise, you are tensing all the muscles you have control over. As you do this, many of the involuntary muscles of your body are also caught up in the squeezing process. When you release the muscles, everything is released in a wave. The contrast between the extreme tension and the resulting relaxation can be very pronounced and give your body a warm, energized feeling. This exercise can break through the hard shell of tension that encases it.

SHAKE

The Shake exercise is probably the simplest and most profound Zen Yoga exercise. It gives you instant, tangible evidence of the potential energy you have, literally, at your fingertips. It can be done anytime, anywhere...and feels great.

To begin, stand with your feet shoulder-width apart. Hold your arms in front of you, bent at the elbow and relaxed. Your palms are face down. Imagine your hands are covered with water and you simply want to shake it off. Begin slowly and then gradually increase speed as you continue the back-and-forth motion. Feel as if all the tension in your hands is being shaken off. Be sure to keep them loose and relaxed. Shake, shake, shake.

Next, start shaking them up and down vigorously, and then in a side-to-side motion, opening the wrist joints. Next, try rotating them in a circle and then reverse the motion, all the while keeping them loose and relaxed. Finally, return to the natural shaking motion and allow the elbow and upper arms to get involved. Raise your arms over your head and shake. Hold your arms out to the side and shake. Your hands and arms should feel like wet noodles.

Continue the exercise for at least one minute, more if you are able. When you are ready to stop, drop your arms straight down to your sides. Close your eyes and take three long deep breaths. Bring your mind's attention to the tips of your fingers. You should feel a tingling sensation there. This is the rich, oxygenated, and energized blood flowing into your hands. Does it feel good? Imagine that feeling coursing through your whole body. How could debilitating problems such as arthritis or carpal tunnel syndrome have a chance to take hold with such energy flowing through your hands?

Breath Walking simply means linking the bodily movement of walking to your breathing. It is an exercise that may seem quite easy at first, but when you actually try it, you will find that it takes patience and a serious commitment. The reason is that Breath Walking is about slowing down the pace of life, something which most people find alien. But it is of the utmost importance to set aside time to practice some meditative exercise. However difficult it may be, slowing down is imperative for all who seek to identify their spiritual essence and make contact with their inner self.

Breath Walking can be thought of as a method of moving meditation. Some people find sitting meditation too tedious or uncomfortable. Breath Walking offers the alternative of achieving the same mental awareness and concentration while moving the body.

The key to Breath Walking is to really go very slowly. It is very easy to want to rush through this exercise, but it is important to take your time. If you have time constraints, this exercise is best left for another occasion.

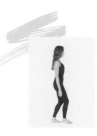

Breath Walking is walking while slowing the rate of your breathing and then walking at the pace of your breathing. It is also another method of connecting the physical body with the mind. As I have said before, when the mind and the body are coordinated, you are able to explore your deeper self. You should find that when you focus on your breathing during Breath Walking, it naturally becomes slower. As a result Breath Walking is very slow and peaceful. When practicing Breath Walking try to slow your breathing down by lengthening both your inhalation and your exhalation.

There are two Breath Walking exercises, Heel to Toe and Thin Ice.

HEEL TO TOE

Heel to Toe Breath Walking is accomplished by simply choosing a distant target and walking toward it by placing the heel of one foot directly in front of the big toe of the other foot. Each step only takes you the length of one foot. Concentrate on your breathing. It is not a race or a competition. Step by step, this exercise offers the illusion of doing something, but as with the Tao, it is really about *not* doing. Indeed, the steps are so small your mind may rebel at doing such a silly exercise, but that is the point. The rebellious mind succumbs to the simple-mindedness of the exercise and finally focuses on the slowness and the breathing. Keep your attention focused. Inhale as you lift your foot, exhale as you place your foot down. Take your time.

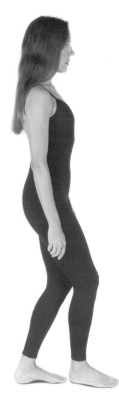

Once you have reached your destination, remain facing the same way and proceed to walk backwards in the same manner, placing the toe of the foot at the heel of the other foot. Again, take your time. Inhale as you lift your foot and exhale as you place it down. Be sure to touch your toe to your heel with each step.

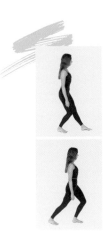

THIN ICE

Thin Ice Breath Walking is much more involved. Each step has two parts coinciding with the inhalation and exhalation of breath.

To begin, stand with your feet shoulder-width apart and take a few long, deep, slow breaths. Once you are relaxed and prepared, begin inhalation and slowly shift your body weight over your left foot. Sink down as you shift your weight. Starting with the heel, pick up your right foot and bring it forward, retaining all your weight back over the left leg. Lightly touch the ground with your right heel. There should be no weight on it, as if you were checking for thin ice on a spring pond. As you begin exhalation, slowly transfer the weight to your right leg flattening your foot down until all the weight is on it. The next inhalation begins as you pick up the left heel and begin to bring the knee up and forward for the next step. The weight remains on the right leg this time as you move your left foot. Exhalation begins as you slowly transfer your weight forward.

It helps to imagine that the ice may break at any moment and you want to be sure of the footing beneath your front foot before transferring your weight to it. Linking the inhalation with each step is the key to this exercise. Breathe in as you place the foot. Breathe out as you shift your weight. The mind is forced to concentrate on the breath and the step at the same time.

Do it slowly. Rushing through this exercise is pointless. Try to practice it for twenty steps.

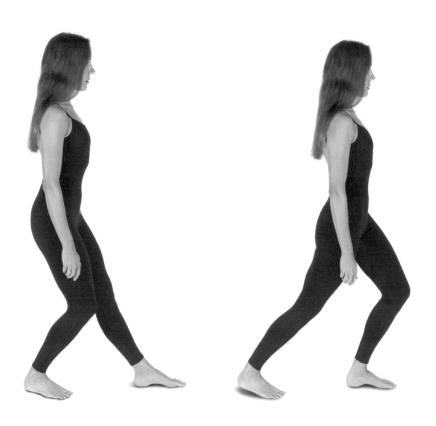

C H A K R A   F O C U S

Chakra Focus consists of simple stillness and breathing meditation exercises. By placing yourself in each posture and focusing your attention on the indicated chakra, you enable your mind to unwind. As you begin to concentrate on your breathing, you activate the power of the chakra and enable a smooth energy flow along the meridians of the body. The deep, rhythmic breathing connects you to the chakra. Before doing these exercises, review the relevant chakra as described in Part 1 to be sure you draw the full meaning from it. Try to maintain each chakra position for at least ten deep breaths.

These exercises can be practiced from either sitting or lying-down positions. I have included both. Use whichever feels best for you.

ROOT FOCUS

■ Sitting

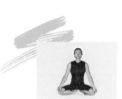

Start in the basic sitting position (page 67), sitting on the floor with your legs bent at the knees and pulled in to your body. Keep each leg flat on the floor. Do not rest one leg on top of the other. Pull one foot into your body so that the heel of the foot is touching the *huyin* point of the root chakra center at the base of the spine. Bring the other foot in to support the first foot. Place a cushion, pillow, or rolled-up towel underneath your buttocks so that your hips are tilted slightly forward. Your knees should be lower than your hips and pointing toward the floor. Don't worry if you cannot get into the exact position at first. This is a long process. Do what you are able and let your body learn.

Sit calmly and quietly for ten deep breaths. Concentrate all of your energy on the root center of your being. Feel yourself physically grounded. The breath should be strong and powerful as you fill your body with oxygen and energy. Feel it rise up through the center of your being.

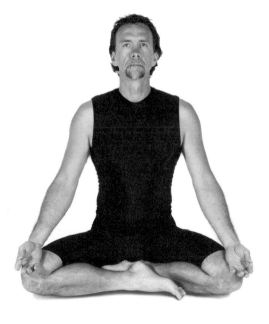

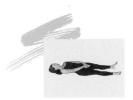

■ Lying down

Lying on your back with your feet naturally flopped apart, place your hands, palms down, over your root chakra center above the pelvis. Remain in position for ten deep breaths. Concentrate all of your energy on the root center of your being. Feel yourself physically grounded. The breath should be strong, powerful and deep as you fill your body with oxygen and energy. Feel it rise up through the center of your being. Hold for ten breaths.

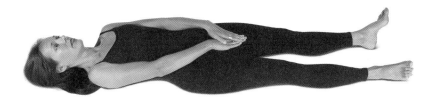

ABDOMINAL FOCUS

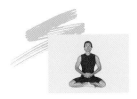

■ Sitting

In the basic sitting position, place your hands palms down over the *dan tien* point of the abdominal chakra center, located three fingers' width below the navel. Begin Basic Abdominal Breathing (page 44) and feel your hands moving in and out with the rhythm of your breath. This muscular action of the abdomen strengthens and tones the whole area as well as massages the internal organs. As you continue this practice, you should begin to feel warmth growing in the chakra area. Allow the feeling to grow strong and expand throughout your body. It is the manifestation of your physical energy and will recharge and energize you. Maintain the position for at least ten breaths.

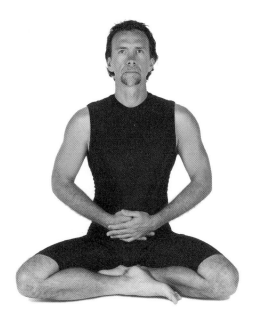

■ Lying down

From a horizontal position, place your hands palms down over the abdominal chakra. Begin deep Abdominal Breathing and feel your hands moving up and down with the rhythm of your breath. Feel the warmth begin to grow in the chakra area. Allow the feeling to grow strong and expand throughout your body. Remain in this position for ten deep breaths.

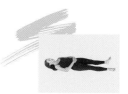

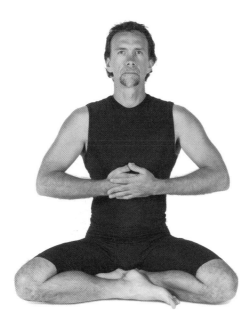

SOLAR PLEXUS FOCUS

■ Sitting

From your basic sitting position, move your hands up to your solar plexus chakra in the center of your torso below the line of your ribs. Focus your attention on the space beneath your hands as you breathe. With each inhalation, push the solar plexus out. The mild resistance from your hands will force the oxygen and energy to flow into all the spaces between the internal organs of the torso. Gently push inward as you breathe out. This intensifies the intrinsic massage of the internal organs and will stimulate energy flow throughout your bodily systems. Maintain the position for ten breaths.

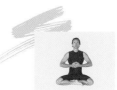

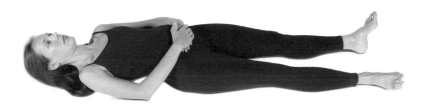

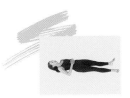

■ Lying down

From a lying-down position, place your hands palms down over the solar plexus chakra. As with the sitting position, feel your hands moving in and out with the rhythm of your breathing. Feel the warmth begin to grow in the chakra area. Allow the feeling to grow strong and expand throughout your body. Remain in position for ten deep breaths.

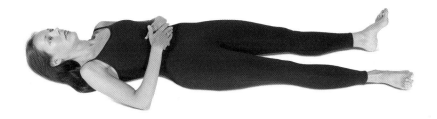

HEART FOCUS

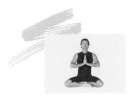

■ Sitting

From your basic sitting position, move your hands up and bring the palms together at your heart center chakra, located at the center of your upper torso at the center point between the nipples. Inhale and raise your chin as you expand your chest. Exhale and bow your head. Bring your lips to your fingertips. Breathe deeply and imagine the energy flowing through your heart, stimulating your emotional being. With each inhalation, feel as if your heart is opening up and love is blossoming. With each exhalation spread that love out to the world. This love is a special energy that grows stronger as you let it flow in and out of you. The more you spread this feeling the stronger it grows. Continue for ten breaths.

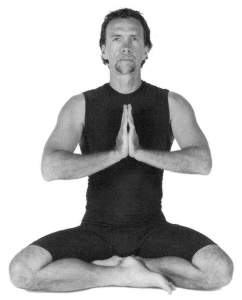

■ Lying down

In a lying-down position, bring your hands together at your heart center chakra. The palms press into each other in a prayer position. The rest of your body should have the feeling of sinking downward into the floor. As with the sitting practice, breathe deeply and feel the energy flowing through your emotional being. With each inhalation, feel as if your heart is opening up and love is blossoming. With each exhalation spread that love out to the world. This love is a special energy that grows stronger as you let it flow in and out of you. The more you spread this feeling, the stronger it grows. Continue for ten breaths.

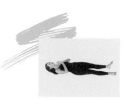

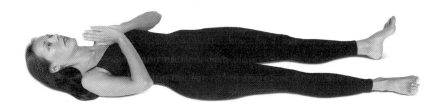

THROAT FOCUS

■ Sitting

From your basic sitting position, move your hands up to your collarbones and trace your fingers inward until you reach the center. Shift your fingers up slightly to find the gap between the bones to find your throat chakra. Breathe deeply and focus the energy into the throat. With each exhalation relax the muscles of the neck and allow the chakra to open wider. As you breathe, feel as if the higher being that resides within you is growing stronger. Hold for ten breaths.

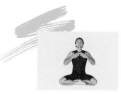

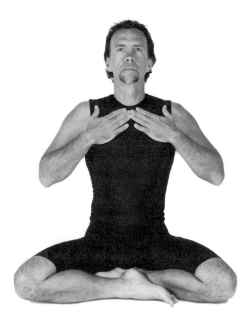

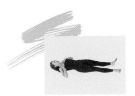

■ Lying down

In a horizontal position, raise your hands to your collarbones and trace your fingers inward until you reach the center. Shift your fingers up slightly to find the gap between the bones to find your throat chakra. Drop your elbows to the floor, and release any excess tension in your arms and chest. Breathe deeply, but concentrate on the higher being within you. Maintain the position for ten breaths.

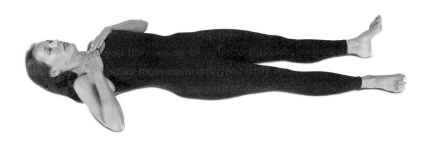

THIRD-EYE FOCUS

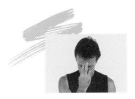

■ Sitting

From your basic sitting position, raise one hand to your forehead and place the tips of the first two fingers on the third-eye chakra, located in the center of the forehead just above the space between the eyebrows. Close your eyes and breathe deeply. Bring all of your attention to the chakra and allow yourself to turn inward

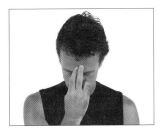

toward the center of your being. Feel your spiritual self growing and expanding outward into the universe. Hold the position for at least ten breaths.

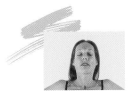

■ Lying down

From your horizontal position on the floor, place a coin the size of a U.S. quarter (about ¾ inch/ 2 cm) on your brow at the third-eye chakra. Close your eyes and begin breathing while maintaining awareness of the subtle sensation of the coin's weight. Use all of your intuitive powers to sense the coin. As time passes, the feeling of the

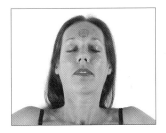

coin will fade. Maintain awareness of the coin for as long as possible. As the feeling fades, your mind will begin to wander. Control it. Keep it focused. Breathe, relax, and let the energy of the universe flow through you. Continue for ten breaths.

CROWN FOCUS

■ Sitting

From your basic sitting position place both hands, palms down, on your crown chakra, on top of your head at the center of the skull. Relax any tension in the shoulders as you breathe and get comfortable in the position. Return to your breathing and allow the inhalation and exhalation to slow as you go deeper into yourself and feel a connection with that which is immortal within you. Maintain the position for at least ten breaths.

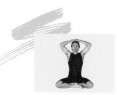

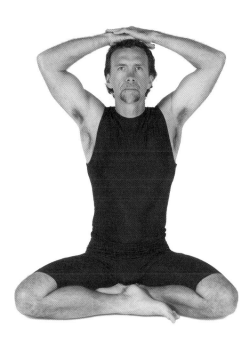

■ Lying down

From a lying-down position, raise your hands over your head and place them, palms down, on your crown chakra, at the top of your head over the center of the skull. Relax your arms and let your elbows rest on the floor. Let your breath lengthen as you draw your awareness into the center of your being, and then follow along as your awareness begins to expand into the universe. Hold for ten breaths.

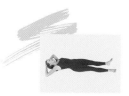

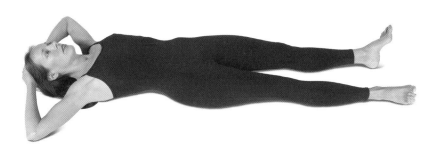

Exercise Summary

In the four exercise chapters we have explored a wide variety of ways to breathe, move, stretch, and relax effectively, ensuring that you are continuously charged with energy. Each of the exercises has the fundamental goal of assisting the flow of energy through your body and helping you to feel happy, healthy, and alive. There should never be anything difficult or strenuous about this practice. Take it slow and steady. In the end, it does not really matter what specific exercise you are doing. The important thing is that you are breathing, moving, and stretching your body while allowing your mind to release, relax, and let go.

The exercises here can be considered opportunities to give yourself what you need to be healthy. While this is by no means a complete list of Zen Yoga exercises, it is a good starting point to give you an idea of the possibilities that exist for helping your body to feel better and your mind to find some measure of peace. Regardless of your body type or fitness level, there are always some types of exercise you can do. Do them. Don't wait until you are "back in shape." Don't wait until you lose a certain number of pounds. *Begin now and do something.* Move your body, stretch your muscles, calm your mind and…remember to BREATHE!

Even if you do nothing else, breathe consciously. This simple practice can change your life. The healthy feelings generated will only make you feel better and better. There is nothing to lose…and everything to gain. Breathe and enjoy!

In the final assessment, it matters only to you what you do for yourself. We each choose how to live our life and must accept the consequences of that behavior. I have found that life is more enjoyable and smoother when your body and mind are working together as allies for you, rather than as enemies fighting against you. It really is common sense, something that seems to be in scarce supply these days. I often hear people admit that they are out of shape and know that they need to start doing "something" to take care of themselves, yet they continue to procrastinate. My comment to them is that there is no time other than right now. This is Zen. Start slowly, do what you need for yourself, take your time…but start *now.*

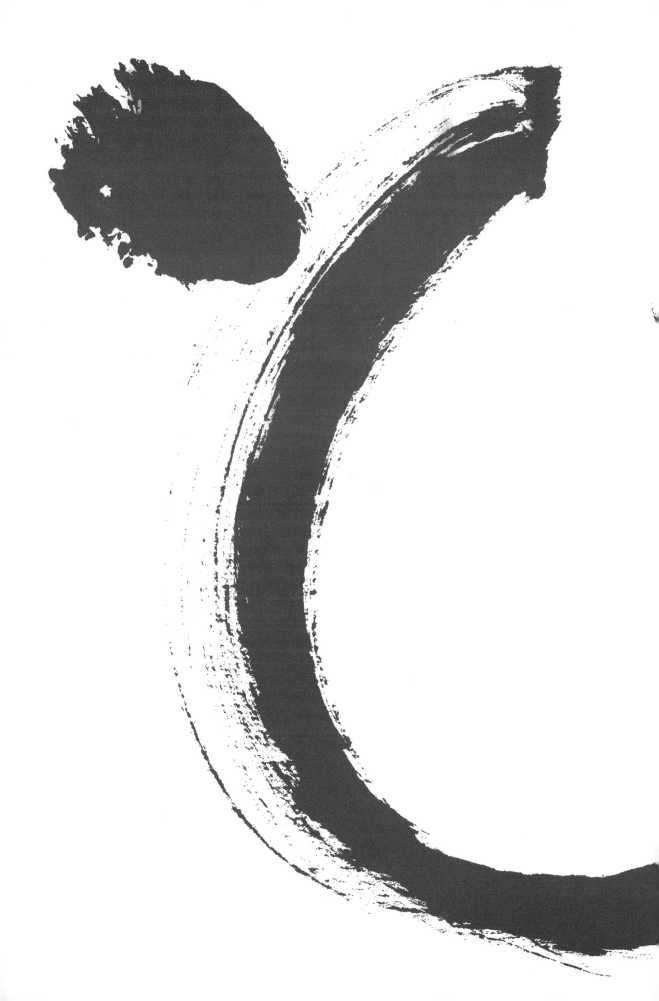

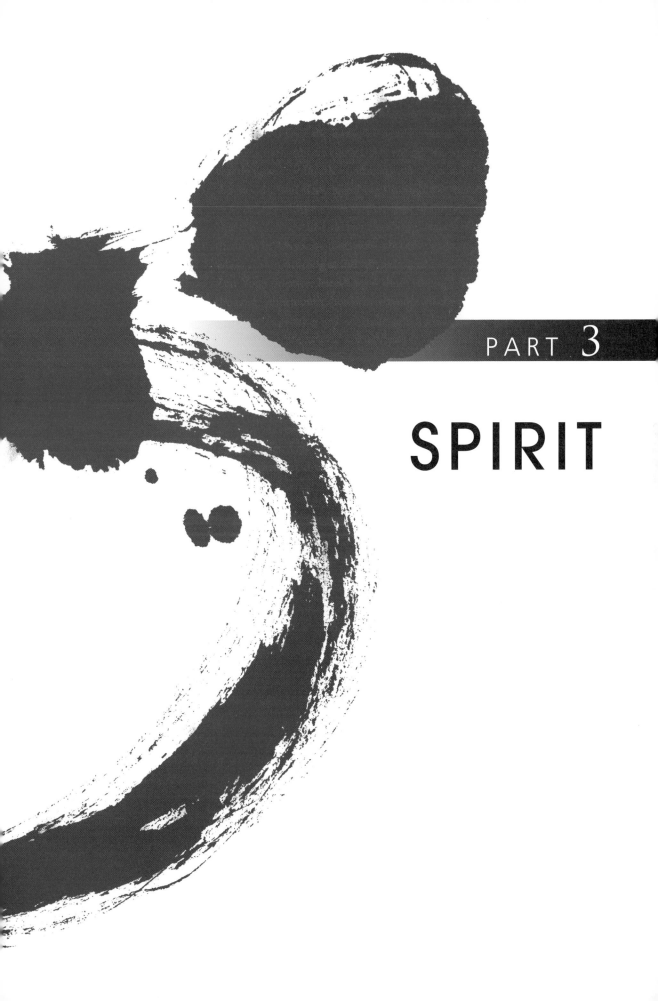

PART 3

SPIRIT

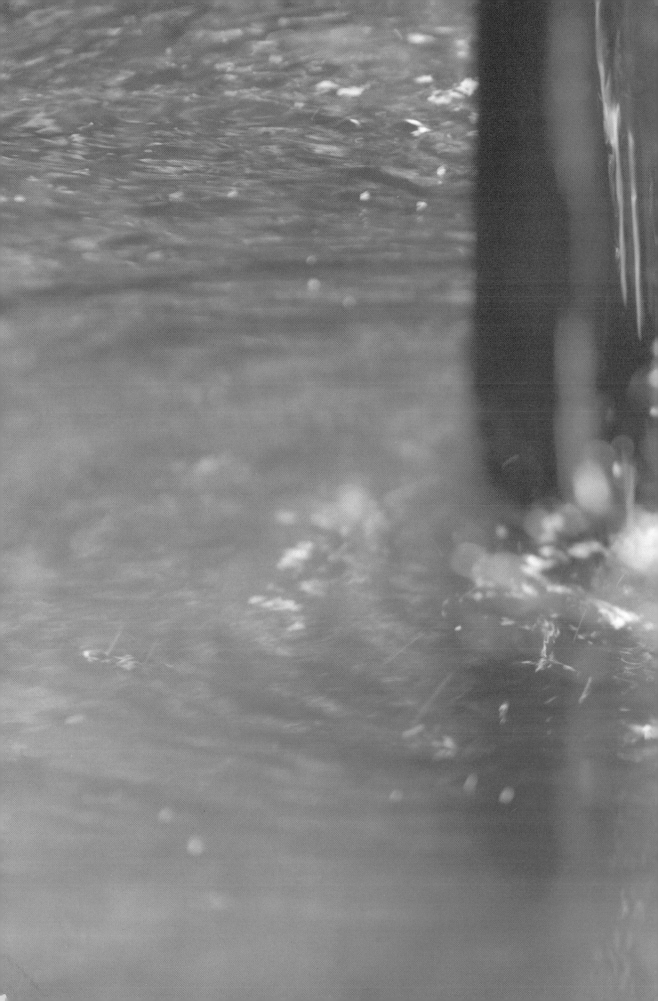

Zen Yoga Spiritual Deepening

What lies behind us and what lies before us
Are tiny matters compared to
What lies within us.

—Ralph Waldo Emerson

The Nature of Spirit

Namaste.   "The divine in me greets the divine in you."

—Hindu greeting

We each have our own concept of what, exactly, the soul or spirit is. For some, their spirituality is faith-based and deeply religious. For others, it is more emotional and based on feelings of the heart. Still others find their spirituality in commune with nature or through extreme sports or other activities. Whatever differences people have in defining the soul or spirit, it is not really in doubt that we are made up of something more than just a physical body and the thought process we call the mind. We have all been able, at times, to step away from our thoughts and feelings and observe ourselves in a larger context. But who is the observer in such instances?

There has to be someone or something there, behind the mask, observing all of life's silliness in which we become entangled. I believe it is a deeper aspect of one's self. Some call this the true self. This deeper aspect of self can manifest itself in many ways. It can be a feeling of knowing things we have never learned, or an understanding of things we have never encountered. It can be a feeling of connection to the world around us. Or it can be a sensing of some higher power that seems to watch over us. Whatever it is, we have a sense of something within us that makes us special and unique, something we can appropriately identify as our spirit.

Actually defining spirit is difficult, because no definition can come close to the truth. Some attempt, however, at definition can help set you on the path toward greater awareness of it. From my personal perspective, I would define the spirit as the state of being totally conscious, alive, and aware. When you are living life and experiencing it at every moment, you are touching your spirit.

This concept is not new. Bhagwan Shree Rajneesh, one of India's most widely respected spiritual teachers, calls it "aliveness." It is a feeling independent of any outward forces. It is being happy without having a reason to be happy. The difficulty lies in reaching this state of being and experiencing it. It is easy to speak of it. Living it is another story.

Lao Tsu, one of China's foremost philosophers, in his work *Tao-te Ching,* observed that plants, animals, and humans are born supple and soft, yet when they die they are stiff and brittle. In order to experience the kind of aliveness to which Lao Tsu and Rajneesh are referring, we must be a disciple of life and allow its soft and supple aspects to prevail. That which is hard and stiff will be broken. Fighting against the natural flow of life will only lead to difficulty and disaster. It is not the way.

Becoming more aware of our spiritual nature is a natural progression for us as human beings. We hunger for more. As we grow and develop, we learn that the pursuit of material possessions is not enough. We begin to crave answers to certain questions about our existence. What are we doing here? What path should we take? What is the purpose? And yet our search always leads back to the same place...deep within the self. The answers to these questions often require some relatively profound thought. By taking time to contemplate things about your life and existence you are facilitating your own spiritual deepening process. Unfortunately, that is a tall order in the chaos of modern life.

SPIRITUAL HEARTBURN

Eating too much too fast is a good way to upset your stomach. The same analogy can be used for how experiences affect our deeper self. We gobble up experiences these days, swallowing them whole, and then stuff in more. We have to buy this new thing, go to that special place, watch this new TV show, do this, be that, and eat, eat, eat...until our lives are filled with a continuous stream of things we hope will fulfill us—or at least fill us up. As these undigested experiences accumulate, our lives become little more than a list of things we have done. Ultimately, we set ourselves up for what I call spiritual heartburn. The spiritual nature that exists within us all is never allowed the peace and quiet it requires to develop into the being we each have the potential to become. Instead it is buried under all the other things. Despite being full, we remain hungry or unfulfilled.

Continuing with the eating analogy, if we learn to slow down our consumption and regulate our eating habits, the digestive system can more easily cope with what we are taking in. Things will be processed better and we will feel healthier.

The same can be said for our spiritual self. When we learn to slow down and experience life at a more natural pace, we find that things don't need to be as hectic or as hard to manage as we may have imagined. We also find that we can focus our attention more completely on whatever we are dealing with, since slowing down the pace at which we do things enables us to see life with greater clarity. We grow calmer and begin to feel increasingly alive.

These days, a great deal of emphasis is put on doing things as quickly as possible. But making life faster does not necessarily make it better, especially when we seem to be rushing toward something we don't perceive clearly or understand. In the past, people spent many years practicing an art or skill. Nowadays, it seems that if you can't learn something in the space between the commercials, it is not worth learning. It's become too much trouble. However, learning to experience the fullness of your life in this present moment should be your prime imperative. The future will be here soon enough. There is no point in rushing to get there, especially since you may not find what you expect when you arrive. Slow down and live in the present. Whatever is going to happen in the future will happen. Deal with it when it gets here.

Zen Yoga training embodies the path to achieving this state of being. Breathing, moving, stretching, and relaxing are the keys to slowing the pace of life and enjoying what you are doing in the magic of the present moment. Whatever the future holds, you will be prepared to experience it fully and be ready to open up to your true self and to your place in the grand adventure. Then your whole being will be ready to coalesce into the manifestation of your spiritual self. When that happens, you won't need any book to tell you what to do.

Experiential Zen Yoga

If you don't feel it, you'll never get it.

—Goethe

One of the things you can do to help yourself feel more in tune with your spiritual nature is to incorporate the Eastern philosophical traditions from part one into your daily life. The chakras, chi energy, yin and yang, the five elements, the eight limbs of yoga, and the Tao are tools to assist you in discovering more about your spiritual nature. They are only mysterious if you don't understand them. Go back and read that section again and contemplate their meanings as they pertain to your life and personal experiences. Examine them, too, according to the value they have for you as you pursue mastery of the concepts and practices of Zen Yoga.

The Eastern traditions have their roots in strong philosophical principles. By learning and understanding the philosophical foundations on which the principles are based, you are able to internalize the concepts and significantly enrich their meaning. But experiencing the principles takes you even deeper, allowing you to internalize them more fully and make each one an integral part of your life. At that point you will have reached your own pinnacle, and you will never again be the same.

EXPERIENCING THE CHAKRAS

Experiencing the chakras is about connecting the mind to the body. They are the sacred places within the body. Opening the chakras and allowing the life force to flow freely through them makes the body and mind stronger while enhancing the spirit. The chakras affect our physical existence, our emotional state of mind, and our spiritual development. Good health and a general state of well-being are the natural result of clear and open chakras. Keeping them infused with energy is of great benefit. In the last chapter, we learned ways to relax by practicing breathing exercises while focusing on the individual chakras. These exercises are an invaluable tool for bringing your mind and body together with your spiritual self. In addition, Microcosmic Orbit breathing is the method for circulating the energy through the chakras. Regular practice of these exercises will bring profound results.

Try to become aware of the different chakras as you go about your daily life. Practice focusing on a certain one and try to bring the principles and feelings of that chakra into your awareness of the body and mind connection. See if you can become aware of things happening within you at a deeper level.

This practice is not easy and can take a long time to produce results, but you will be strengthening the connections inside you and leading the energy to a wonderful place.

EXPERIENCING CHI

Experiencing chi is about becoming aware of the energy of the universe and how you interact with it. As I explained in the section on breathing, conscious breathing allows you to access that energy and use it effectively. Using the breath to direct the chi through your body along the meridians and into each of the chakras is the best way to give the body what it needs to be happy and healthy. Chi is vital to life. Chi is life. Natural, conscious breathing is a method of tapping into the life force of chi. It opens the floodgates of existence and encourages a continuous transfer or exchange of energy between you and the universe. When you do this, you are able to build up the body's intrinsic power. The Shake exercise followed by the Energy Ball Qigong exercise are the quickest and simplest ways to feel the energy flowing through you and the best method to generate reserves of chi for your body to use. Practice them daily and you will experience your chi.

EXPERIENCING YIN AND YANG

Experiencing yin and yang is about bringing balance into your life. In the chapter on Zen Yoga fundamentals, I discuss the importance of balance in the universe. Learning to bring balance into your life is a key aspect of deepening your spirituality. By taking a more practical look at balance and relating it to your physical Zen Yoga training, you can gain a tangible understanding of how balance affects you.

A number of the exercises in this book (Zen Yoga Balance, Inversions, Tension Release) help in the process of incorporating the principle of yin and yang into training. By experiencing contrasting feelings and sensations, you are able to strengthen that connection.

The first step in incorporating yin and yang into your life is learning how to become more acutely aware of when things are out of balance. Only when you realize a problem exists can you take measures to rectify it.

Becoming aware of your balance throughout your daily travels allows you to feel the continuity of your spiritual life. This awareness connects you to the natural flow of the universe. Life has its own pace and rhythm. Trying to control it is like trying to catch a river with a bucket; it is easy to become overwhelmed. There is a time for being in motion and a time for being at rest. If you are trying to move when you should be resting, you are fighting against the natural flow of things. By balancing yourself, you learn to allow things to take their course and let your life travel with the flow. You may often hold on too tight when letting go might be the better way to reach your goal.

One of the most important principles embodied by the concept of yin and yang, is the relationship between stillness and motion. During daily life we are in constant motion. We imagine we are motionless at night when we sleep, but we do not actually experience stillness when we are unconscious. And if we are awake in bed we are, more often than not, tossing and turning, trying to get comfortable or worrying about yesterday or tomorrow. True stillness is rarely experienced. Stillness is the natural state before movement begins, and yet it is also the basis of all movement.

Understanding the symbiosis of stillness and movement can guide you in establishing true balance and control within yourself. The best method for learning the principle embodied in stillness is to be still—completely still.

Pick a position, standing, sitting or lying down. When first starting this exercise it is probably best to be lying down to reduce the fatigue placed on the muscles. Once in position, do not move at all. The goal is to achieve total, pure stillness. This is different from what we normally think of as being still or quiet, in which some motion, no matter how miniscule, is inevitable. The point here is to make absolutely no movement whatsoever. No adjustment, no shifting of weight, no scratching, nothing. Once you have achieved stillness, relax the focus of your eyes and bring your attention inward to your abdominal chakra. Begin to practice Abdominal Breathing. Keep completely still in every other way. Ignore the itch on your cheek, the twinge in your foot, and any aches in your muscles. Once you breathe in and fill your lungs, stop. Freeze completely. Stop everything. The beating of your heart should be the only sensation. This is true stillness. Try this again when you breathe out.

This may seem an oversimplification, but if you practice it enough you will eventually come to understand the difference between absolute stillness and what usually passes for it. You will become intimately aware of each muscle that is in use. And when you finally do move, the movement initiated from this stillness will be done with complete awareness and true intent and will reflect a perfect union of mind and body.

Practicing this stillness exercise offers a vivid demonstration of the role meditation can play in helping you relax.

EXPERIENCING THE FIVE ELEMENTS

Experiencing the five elements is about recognizing the cycle of life and how it relates to you individually and the experiences that make you who you are. The elements affect each other in a continuous process.

The elements themselves can be thought of as symbols to describe how everything in the world relates to everything else. An analogy can be made between the features and actions of something, and the characteristics of the five elements. The properties of things that are similar to those of wood are classified as wood, those similar to fire, as fire, etc. Points on the compass, for instance, can be classified according to the five elements. East is classified as wood because the ascending characteristics of wood are similar to the sunrise. South is classified as fire because the heat of fire is similar to the warmth found in the south (by those in the northern hemisphere). West is classified as metal because the descending characteristics of metal are similar to the sunset. North is classified as water because the coldness of water is similar to the cold found in the north (again, by those in the northern hemisphere). Finally, the center is classified as earth because it is the balance or neutrality of the directions, the reference point.

Overabundance

Becoming aware of the natural cycle that exists within all things allows you to see the world more clearly. Learning to balance the five elements helps to align the energy of your environment in order to create an atmosphere that is conducive to your obtaining access to your maximum energy. If you can learn to recognize when there is an overabundance of one or more of the elements within yourself, you will be able to address this imbalance.

■ Overabundance of wood

An overabundance of wood can lead to inconsistency or lack of assertiveness in daily life. This typically manifests itself as something that starts with an overzealous beginning and is eventually dropped or left unfinished. It is a state of the will growing weak. You find yourself becoming too passive, so that apathy takes over. Other times you may find yourself becoming too dependent on the actions of others. There is a tendency toward laziness and procrastination, doing only just enough to get by. If this describes you, then you have an overabundance of wood.

To reverse this problem, work to gain control of yourself. Finish projects you start. Make decisions without waiting for others to take the initiative. Assert yourself and shake off the lethargy.

■ Overabundance of fire

An overabundance of fire can lead to a lack of sensitivity and compassion toward others. There is a tendency to be forceful and impulsive, to drive through your agenda without a care for anyone else's thoughts or feelings. There often seems to be an underlying impatience with everything. This impatience can lead to frustration, which, in turn, builds until there is an emotional outburst. If this describes you, then you have an overabundance of fire.

To reverse this problem, step back. Take notice of others around you and see if your actions are disturbing them. Too often you may be unaware that your behavior is disruptive. Relax. There is no need for everything to be done immediately, exactly as you want. Allow the possibility that there may be another way of doing things.

■ Overabundance of earth

An overabundance of earth can lead to getting stuck in a rut of your own making. There is a disinterest in any type of excitement or adventure. In fact, you have little interest in much of anything. Sometimes in this state, fear of the unknown can lead to a simple fear of the new. However, if you attempt nothing new, then you will miss the enriching experience of the new. You begin to second-guess yourself as you lose faith in your intuition. If this describes you, then you have an overabundance of earth.

To reverse this problem, seek out change. Do something to shock yourself out of your routine. Don't be afraid to fail. Even if you don't succeed, you will become stronger for having put in the effort. Do something different, right now.

■ **Overabundance of metal**

An overabundance of metal can lead to an aggressive thirst for power or wealth. There is an underlying aggressiveness to all of your undertakings. You may become unreasonable and inflexible as you drive toward your goal, driven by a continuous desire for more and more, a thirst that cannot be quenched. If this describes you, then you have an overabundance of metal.

To reverse this problem, stop accumulating things. Be generous. Start by giving something of value away to someone. In these times it is fine to be autonomous and pioneering, but don't cut yourself off from your humanity. Learn the meaning of compassion and humility.

■ **Overabundance of water**

An overabundance of water can lead to moodiness and depression. There is a tendency to become deeply immersed in your own issues. You find yourself in a place that is very insular as you begin to shun contact with others. Your behavior can often become subjective and unpredictable even though your circumstances are unchanged. If this describes you, then you have an overabundance of water.

To reverse this problem, get out and meet new people. Start a new hobby. Do something that takes you out of your little box and lets you interact with the world. Everyone you meet is an opportunity to learn something new and different. Take a chance, smile.

EXPERIENCING THE EIGHT LIMBS OF YOGA

Experiencing the eight limbs of yoga is about commitment to a positive lifestyle. The ideas embodied in the principle of the eight limbs of yoga constitute guidelines for living in a manner which helps keep your spiritual essence clean and virtuous. It is a method for allowing it to fully develop. Bring the eight limbs into your life with the intention of using them to help you complete yourself.

The *yama*, or abstentions, are ways of remaining true to your self. By maintaining a lifestyle of basic goodness, there is no room for negative forces to take hold and grow. As you become more spiritual, you will find yourself naturally manifesting goodness and generating positive energy. The *yama* seem obvious when we first look at them, but it takes effort to maintain them when things become difficult. There is a tendency to believe that it is impossible to adhere to the *yama*, but if you maintain your integrity and try your best, the energy of the universe will tend to flow in that direction and you will find it easier to maintain them.

The *niyama*, or observances, are ways of creating a strong sense of self. While the *yamas* are things to avoid, the *niyama* are things to cultivate within yourself. By learning the *niyama* life skills that keep you growing and developing, you will create harmony within yourself and continue on the path toward realizing your perfection. The *niyama* can be intimidating, but with contemplation you will find their truth.

The *asana*, or postures, are ways of building a strong body. Moving and stretching are the primary concerns of the physical body. By strengthening and developing the muscles of the body, you will find it much easier to maintain a healthy lifestyle. It is an upward spiral. Do something every day, and each day you will grow stronger throughout your life.

The *pranayama*, or breathing, is your connection to the energy of the universe. It is the fundamental dimension of human existence. When you stop breathing, life is over. Practice breathing with quality and make each breath a special event. This simple practice can change your life if you give it the opportunity.

The *pratyahara*, or introspection, is bringing the mind under control. It is the reigning in of the frantic thoughts that keep you distracted. As you begin to discover yourself through introspection or meditation, you will start to think more deeply about who you are and what your purpose is. Don't shy away from these thoughts. Explore them and work to discover your inner self. Don't be afraid; fear is often only a defense mechanism that your mind puts up to keep you from discovering the secrets of your true self.

The *dharana* is deep concentration, a meditation on the thoughts that arise from within. We cannot just push the thoughts aside. Instead we need to accept them and understand where they came from. Understanding who you are is a natural progression. Your purpose in this life becomes clear only when you can go beyond the mundane world and reach deep within yourself and experience the energy that is flowing through you. Only after you feel this energy will you be able to begin directing its flow.

The *dhyana* is the pure awareness of existence. It is the directed focus of the mind on the essence of your being. When you find that glowing seed, you are able to understand that the seed makes you unique and yet it also connects you with everything in the universe. Understanding this duality in being both a separate entity and part of the complete whole is a profound step in your personal evolution.

The *samadhi*, or enlightenment, is the final step. It is when you go beyond the trials and tribulations of daily life that you finally realize your perfection and become aware of your existence both as an individual spiritual entity and as an integrated part of the grand scheme of things.

Then you will be ready to begin.

EXPERIENCING THE TAO

At its most basic, experiencing the Tao is about existing fully in the present moment. It is enjoying life regardless of the circumstances. Have you ever met people who are unhappy with their situation and continuously gripe that if only they could change this or that they would be happy, or who feel that if they lived somewhere else or had a different father or mother things would be better? Unfortunately, a darkness within is not cured by moving the body from one place to another. Chances are they would be just as miserable if they got the change they were looking for.

Living the Tao is about finding the freedom to enjoy whatever you have at this moment. True freedom is adapting to the infinite variety of life's conditions without losing confidence in your ability to connect to the deeper spiritual essence within.

This philosophy is based on simple propositions. If you have no expectations, then almost everything that happens is a surprising success. If you have no desires, then everything pleasant you experience is a bonus.

This is Zen, the true meaning of following the Tao. It is being alive in the present moment, experiencing life as it happens, and reacting to it in a calm and natural way. It is living fully and completely.

Start today. Look at the plants and animals around you. The essence of life is everywhere, in everything. All the things that happen to you are part of the flow of energy in the universe. If you are constantly having difficulty, you need to stop and carefully examine the way you are living. Is it possible that you are fighting against the flow? We all have times of stress or hardship, but everything that happens to us is an opportunity for learning and growing in some respect. It may be painful or difficult but, at least in this view, there is a benefit that comes from all the problems. Relax and take the time to observe things as they are, especially when you cannot control them. Allow things to take their course and happen naturally. And, of course, pay attention to the present moment. Then you will be well on the journey to freeing your spiritual nature.

Cultivating Quietism

In moments of insight,
we become aware of a connection to nature.

—Colin Wilson

Quietism is a form of Taoist meditation. As I explained in chapter 2, it is a state of mind that results from letting the thoughts in your mind sink down, leaving the mind clear and pure. Imagine a glass of water with a handful of dirt swirling around in it. If you set that muddy water aside, eventually the dirt will sink to the bottom and the water will become clear. With quietism, you set your mind aside and allow the thoughts to settle down.

For the most part the mind is not used to being peaceful. It can't be turned off and on again like a light switch. When the mind does actually calm down, we are too ready to turn immediately to some new distraction. With quietism, we let all of that go and just exist. As I have noted often in this book, the nature of the life we lead makes it increasingly imperative that we find a peaceful place and set aside time to stop and breathe for a few moments every day. If we recall the principle of yin and yang, the loud and busy part of daily life needs to be balanced with peace and quiet in order to bring you back into harmony with yourself. Cultivating quietism is the way to reach that balance, which we do in the context of a deeper experience with nature. An integral relationship with nature is a fundamental dimension of human existence. Without it, we lose our sense of the interconnectedness of all living things. The trees, grass, mountains, oceans, and animals of the world contain the essence of life, and to deny ourselves exposure to them is to deprive ourselves of what we need to be an inherent part of the natural world. At the heart of quietism is an intense experience of our connection with the natural world.

Please note, the intent of quietism is not to clear thoughts entirely from the mind. Instead, it is to focus your thoughts and attention on a natural scene or setting so intensely that your usual patterns of thinking are interrupted or temporarily redirected. You are not attempting to stifle your thoughts, but simply to cultivate a state of such total concentration that the unwanted thoughts cannot successfully intrude or take control of the quiet space you are creating. This is done by focusing your senses on a natural setting and then allowing your thoughts complete freedom to respond.

The first step is to find an environment that is suitable to you. Choose one of those described below in which to immerse yourself, or one from another environment accessible to you. Select whatever sitting position is comfortable and settle in. Begin with your breathing. In this exercise it is not necessary to become overly fixated on your breath. By now you have built up breathing skills that enable you to find the rhythm of breathing appropriate to the situation. Next, begin to observe your chosen environment. Become aware of the colors and sounds. Expand the play of your senses. Relax your eyes and expand your field of vision. Let the sounds wash over you. Breathe and inhale the essence of it. Feel the touch of the wind on your body. Become a part of it.

Below is a list of environments you can use for this exercise. Whichever one you choose, all that is important is that you try to experience the essence or essential nature of it and absorb it into your own sense of being.

ENVIRONMENTS FOR OBSERVATION

Day Sky

The day sky is deep and clear. The clouds bring movement and change. Time slows down as the clouds drift slowly by. Become aware of their subtle movement and change in form as they drift above you. If you imagine each cloud as an occasional intruding thought, let it pass by and move on. Release your mind and let it be free within the vast confines of the sky and all that is there.

Night Sky

The night sky presents the quality of silent eternity. The stars and constellations hint at the vastness of the cosmos. Different stars and constellations appear with the changing seasons. Calmly observe the stars and the moon as they wander across the night sky. The moon embodies a magical strength and mystery. Let the mind expand to fill the heavens, and all other thoughts are quickly and easily let go.

Ocean

The ocean is immense and ever changing. It is continuously moving, yet from a distance appears still. The ocean reflects the mind, deep and mysterious. Let the waves match your breath as they wash onto the shore in a continuous, never ending motion. Listen to the sound of the waves. Let the sound wash over you. Exist within that moment.

Running Water

The continuous movement of running water reflects the mind. Stopping the flow of water is like trying to stop the thoughts of the mind. It is better to simply redirect the thoughts gently rather than fight against the relentless flow. Allow the mind to become like water. Let it flow through your being.

Mountains

Mountains contain the essence of the earth's strength. Feel the massive solidity of a mountain. It cannot be moved. Strength and solidity are deeply embedded in the earth. Allow the mind to be solid as the mountain, unfazed by petty thoughts and emotions. Feel the power.

Trees

The life cycle of a tree reflects the cycle of all life. From seed to sapling to mature tree to dead wood, the tree passes through the cycle as we all do. Each tree is unique and embodies the essence of life. Roots sink deep into the earth. Imagine the wind as a wave of discursive thought. The tree does not fight against the wind, instead it moves with the wind, swaying back and forth allowing the wind to pass through. Bring that feeling within yourself.

Fire

Fire contains warmth and vitality. Yet its erratic and wild movement reflects the mind's penchant for flitting from one thought to another in rapid succession. It is difficult to focus on a single point of flame. Don't focus the eyes; instead, simply let them follow the movement of the flame. Let the mind flow with the dance of the fire. Feel the glow of the fire within you.

Quietism settings can be found anywhere and everywhere. People who live in big cities may often feel that access to natural settings is rare or spoiled. Parks, gardens, and rooftops all offer opportunities to cultivate peace within. Even settings which encompass active urban life can be experienced within the framework of quietism as long as the setting is one that is very familiar to you and in which you feel wholly comfortable and at ease—a local coffee shop, for instance, a library or bookstore, even taking time to sit and watch the family pet can be considered practicing quietism. It may take a leap of imagination but, after all, humans and human artifacts are parts of nature and, properly approached, can offer entry to the quietism we seek.

Take the time to breathe and relax whenever possible. Nature exists all around us; we just rarely experience it. Stop. Breathe. Relax and enjoy it. This practice allows your mind to free itself of its habitual thought patterns and opens up infinite possibilities.

Mindfulness

You must live in the present,
Launch yourself on every wave,
Find your eternity in each moment.

—Henry David Thoreau

By now we understand that the mind has a chronic tendency to distraction. Most of us live life on automatic pilot. Our spiritual nature, the inner essence of who we truly are, has been buried under a mass of constant programming. We travel through life hardly ever noticing how mindless much of it is. There is so much else to do! We juggle ten different things at once and barely stay a step ahead of chaos and collapse. Our attention is split into fragments. We talk on the phone while driving and eat dinner while watching television. This mindless multitasking actually seems to work. We get everything done, but the price we pay in our physical well-being and mental health can be exorbitant and won't be noticed until it is too late.

The acquisitiveness that infuses our value system results in the obsessive collection of experiences and the ridiculous accumulation of more things. All the while, our inner being withers from inattention. We think if we get *that*, we will be happy. If we go *there*, we will be satisfied. If we do *this*, we will be complete. We develop a multitude of habitual reactions and conditioned responses that lead nowhere. At best we may briefly experience feelings of well-being or inspiration, which still leave us searching for something we can't identify.

That something is *who we are*.

It is awareness...a mindfulness of our inner self and our place in existence.

The cultivation of this kind of mindfulness demands our attention and yet is so simple and so obvious.

How many times, for instance, have you made a mistake and then afterwards thought of simple things you could have done or said to avoid or remedy it? Perhaps you got up too fast and cracked your knee on the coffee table. Or, looking elsewhere, banged your elbow on a doorframe. Or thought of a witty comeback ten minutes after the conversation ended.

Cultivating mindfulness is a method of learning to be in touch with the present moment. It allows us access to all of our knowledge as well as mental and physical skills, whenever we need them, instead of long after the moment has passed. Mindfulness allows us to see things more accurately and relate to the world in a more spontaneous and genuine manner. Mindfulness builds skills to navigate daily life more smoothly.

Modern life can sometimes seem like barely controlled hysteria. Everyone is rushing at breakneck speed in the pursuit of happiness. The truth is that there is no happiness anywhere but in the present moment. This is not to say that there is no happiness in remembering the past or in planning the future—as long as you are mindfully present while doing it. Practicing mindfulness is enabling ourselves to take advantage of every opportunity that comes along to make life genuinely richer, fuller and more enjoyable.

The Japanese word *shoshin* means beginner mind. Whenever we do something for the first time, we have to concentrate on it in order to do it correctly, but as we become skilled at it, we soon stop paying attention to the action of doing it because we learn to perform it habitually. In Zen Yoga the practice of *shoshin* means to learn to retain mindfulness even as the task becomes routine. By maintaining a beginner's frame of mind, we keep our attention fixed on the action in the present moment. If we are able to cultivate mindfulness of something that is routine or boring, then it gains a deeper meaning, and the more alive we feel by doing it. The practice of *shoshin* allows mindfulness to become natural and part of our everyday life.

A good example would be washing your car. Basically you have two choices. You can grumble about it and be unhappy the whole time, doing a shoddy job that leaves you unsatisfied and the car marginally clean, *or* you can wash the car as if you have never washed a car before and make sure that every nook and cranny is spotless and magnificent. It will take about the same amount of time to wash it either way, but the first way will leave you as unsatisfied as when you started. In contrast, when you finish washing the car with mindfulness, you have the satisfaction of having experienced living in the moment of washing the car, and the car will be immaculate, since it will reflect the spirit of the effort you put into cleaning it.

This kind of exercise can be done with any chore, such as writing a report, washing dishes, cooking dinner, mowing the lawn, or doing laundry. Any task that seems mundane can be made special by being done mindfully. Even simple actions such as climbing the stairs or opening a door are opportunities to be mindful. If you are going to allocate the time to performing a task, why not offer the mind the opportunity to experience it as well? That may sound rather difficult, but just trying to do so will be enlightening. By seeking to make everything you do a reflection of your mindful self, you enhance the quality of life and hone the awareness of your mind.

One method for cultivating *shoshin* mindfulness in Zen Yoga practice is to learn to do simple, everyday tasks in a completely new or different way. Our daily living is filled with unconscious and mechanical behavior. We are not mindful of these habits because they have become…well, habits. In order to cultivate mindfulness in these situations, we need to challenge ourselves to become more fully aware of what we are doing. For instance, how many ways can you think of to open a door, take your seat at a restaurant, or greet someone you meet everyday in mundane circumstances?

CHANGE HANDS

For most people, one hand is more dominant than the other. You have spent your whole life doing certain things with that dominant hand, such as brushing your teeth, throwing a ball, combing your hair, and writing. Doing some of these simple things with the other hand is quite difficult. Try to brush your teeth with the other hand. It is not as easy as you might think. You actually have to pay attention to what you are doing. This is a moment of *shoshin*, the beginner's mind. When brushing your teeth with your dominant hand, no concentration is needed. You are free to let your mind wander off, mindless. *Shoshin* brings you into the present moment.

See if you can incorporate this mindfulness practice into your daily life at some level. Practice simple tasks with the less dominant hand. Break the habitual actions and train yourself to become aware of what you are doing.

MOMENTS OF MINDLESSNESS

We have all done it. Dropped or spilled something, lost the keys, broken the glass or even banged into the edge of the table for the umpteenth time. Training yourself to be mindful helps you avoid these things. When the mind is calm and aware, you perceive the world around you more clearly. You think faster and react faster. You know where you are, where you are going, and what you are going to do when you get there. Yet there will be lapses. Treat them as opportunities to pay attention and learn.

If you have a moment of mindlessness, don't make a big deal of it; treat it as a choice. You can sit there getting angry, fuming, rubbing your elbow, berating yourself for not being mindful, and then eventually go back to being mindful; *or* you can acknowledge the fact that you were mindless for a moment and go back to being mindful. Skip the self-pity or self-blame... it's not that important.

Once you choose to take the path of cultivating mindfulness, all the troubles life throws at you become training material. Learn from your moments of mindlessness. Let them teach you about yourself.

And be sure not to confuse thinking about mindfulness with true mindfulness. Thinking about being in the present moment is not being in the present moment.

In the final analysis, it is not really about actually being mindful.

It is simply about being.

Spiritual Skills

The only thing permanent about our behaviors is our belief that they are so.

—Moshe Feldenkrais

As you continue the process of deepening the awareness of your spirituality, it is useful to develop the skills that will assist you along the way. Patience, peacefulness and the ability to live a normal life are simple and effective ways of helping yourself become who you truly are. During your daily life, take time to reflect on how the philosophy and principles of Zen Yoga affect the world around you. See if you can recognize them in the people you meet and the things you experience. Not only will this process help you to understand them better, it will also embed the practice deeper within you so that it becomes part of your personal existence.

PRACTICING PATIENCE

Tense and stressed-out people believe that rushing from one task to another, one thought to another, is the best way to get things done. Some drive themselves with a competitive force so strong they fail to see that their way of life is little more than a façade around a house of cards. One failure or defeat threatens to bring the whole thing crashing down. Sometimes they prop it up with drugs, alcohol, food, or something else that gives them a sense of control or at least satisfaction. But it is an illusion. Control already has been lost, and they are merely trying to hang on for dear life.

Behind this kind of behavior lies an impatience so pervasive that it destroys concentration and puts the person at risk both physically and mentally. For many it is a downward spiral toward disaster. In Zen Yoga training, we seek to reverse this spiral through breathing, moving, stretching, and relaxing. Living mindfully in the present moment allows us to experience the flow of life differently. But this takes patience, without which we live in a state of distorted perceptions and unfulfilled expectations.

But how does one consciously cultivate patience?

Try these simple practices:

- Make a conscious effort to close your mouth and really listen to what others are saying. Allow them to finish their sentences, then take a deep breath and respond to what they said. Do not talk about yourself or how what they are talking about relates to you. Try to focus on what they said and relate your response to their experience. See if you can get a sense of what they really are trying to tell you.

- Blunt your sharp edges. See if you can pause before you react to an unpleasant event before your autopilot reaction takes over. Force yourself to take three deep breaths before you yell or lash out. Do not allow trivial things to get under your skin.

- Loosen the knots within you. Soften your stance on things. Sometimes other people have points to make that are as valid as your own. Take a deep breath and reflect on their needs. You do not have to win every argument. Concede their position and see what results. Surprisingly, you often get much more than you expected.

- Let the dust settle. There is no need to cultivate conflict. Take a deep breath and look inward. Is the conflict you seek within you? Why let it take hold?

- Put into practice the principles of Zen Yoga as I have discussed them in this book.

- Enjoy life more, fret less.

GO FOR THE PEACE

Building personal Zen Yoga skills is not a contest or competition. There are no prizes. Every *body* is different as is every mind. Don't expect to be able to do everything at once. It is the *doing* that is important, not what is done or when it is done or how much is done. Zen Yoga helps loosen the mind's control of the body so the body moves of its own accord toward its own end instead of engaging in essentially useless competition or vain efforts at ego reinforcement.

Don't struggle needlessly, stop...surrender. Allow yourself to yield and go with the flow. The magic of real life is in the living.

- Explore gentleness. Things do not always have to be hard and forceful.

- Find the softness in things.

- Do not fear being weak. The only weakness is fear.

- Let things go. Holding on too long stunts development.

- Forgive others. Do not be afraid.

Finding the peace that exists within you is about seeking your spiritual essence and allowing it to grow and flourish. Coupled with the breathing, moving, stretching, and relaxing of Zen Yoga practice, achieving peace is one of the keys to unlocking your true self.

NORMAL LIFE

Many people say they just want a normal life. But actually there is no such thing. There is just life. We cannot spend our time complaining about what could have been. We cannot regret anything. Everything that has come before makes us who we are right now. Looking back to what could have been distracts us from the path that lies before us. We would not be here if we had made other choices. That path is irrelevant.

Pay attention to the path you are on.

Life is an endless challenge. Making choices and overcoming adversity define who we are. Each one of us is an individual, yet we are also part of life as a whole.

As we come to realize our connection to the flow of the Tao, we feel the chi traveling through the chakras. We balance the elements and the yin with the yang. We feel truly alive.

Meet your challenges, face your fears, and live your life. *That's* a life lived well.

Remember to Breathe

The only thing you need to do is breathe;
All the rest will fall into place.

—A. H.

One of the greatest difficulties in teaching the body proper breathing habits is the simple fact that the body doesn't need us to be aware of its breathing in order to function. The challenge then becomes remembering to put what we have learned into practice. Regular, deep, conscious breathing exercises will fill you with energy and make your body feel better. This is indisputable. More oxygen and energy inside your body can only help.

During the typical day there are innumerable opportunities to practice deep breathing. You just need to become more aware of the amount of time that is available in your daily life for breathing. Everyone has spent time sitting in traffic or standing in line at a checkout counter. These are ideal times to devote a few moments to deep breathing. During those moments it is easy to give in to annoyance, to get stressed out. Why not take the opportunity to practice your deep breathing? Whenever there is a pause for a minute or two, you have a choice as to how you will react. You can choose to fret and fume, or you can take some deep breaths and enjoy the moment you are living in. It is your choice.

ATTACHING EVENTS

There are many ways to remind yourself to practice your deep breathing. One of the best methods is to attach breathing practice to an action or event that occurs frequently in daily life. By getting into the habit of associating deep breathing with these events and actually taking one or more breaths before, or as, you engage in them, you begin to train the body to get used to conscious breathing.

Take a deep breath

- before you start eating a meal

- whenever you look at your watch

- before getting out of bed in the morning

- before or after getting into bed at night

- before you start your car

- before and after brushing your teeth

- whenever the phone rings

- Between clicks of the remote

- Each time you pull open a door

- Before serving in tennis or taking a free throw in basketball

The list is endless. There are hundreds of things you do daily that are perfect moments to become aware of your breathing. I encourage you to create a list of your own that will help you form the habit of remembering to breathe at just that moment. Eventually your body will begin to enjoy the feeling and start to want to breathe deeper on its own. Then you will find yourself remembering to breathe at other times of the day. When this happens, fill your life with the happy, healthy feelings that are generated by breathing.

Continuing Journey

Where are you hurrying to?
You will see the same moonlight tonight,
Wherever you go.

—Shikibu Izumi

Experiencing Zen Yoga is not something that you do once and then forget about. Nor is it something you do at a specific time each day or week. Developing a personal Zen Yoga practice is a continuing process of growth. It is a journey inward, a chance for discovering the true perfection that resides within you. Zen Yoga is not something you learn, it is something you are. It is not something about which anyone can say "been there, done that."

The basic precepts of Zen Yoga are simple tenets that should be applied to every aspect of your life, making it more peaceful and enjoyable no matter what you do.

SLOW DOWN

What's your hurry? Life can run at any pace. It is within you to decide how fast to live your life. Rushing through it only gets you to the end quicker. And there are so many wonderful things that you will miss along the way. "Take your time to stop and smell the roses," the old saying goes. It is pertinent here. Don't be a slave to time. Learn to manage it effectively. Let time be an ally, not an enemy. You don't have to get everything done at once. You may not need to get everything done—period.

EXPAND YOUR HEART

We are all on our own journey. Be forgiving and accepting of others. They are simply trying to find their own way in this world. Many are lost and struggling to find answers. Don't judge them; accept them as they are. Offer what you can. By giving, you create an inexhaustible source of positive energy within. Above all, allow yourself to enjoy life without exception. Smile, laugh, dance, skip, and giggle.

NOURISH YOUR BODY

Conscious breathing is the simplest, yet most beneficial thing you can do for yourself. Bringing in oxygen and energy fills the body with the elixir it needs to flourish. Give your body what it needs. It takes very little effort, simply a desire to change your routine and a conscious effort to remember to breathe.

CALM YOUR MIND

Relaxation is more than physical. It is about stilling the torrent of thoughts. Don't let your mind control you. Allow your thoughts to settle and clarity will result. The mind can be a powerful tool when you teach it to follow you, as opposed to you following it—but it needs to be trained. It has had your whole life up until now to run free. It will take time and effort to rein it in. Be patient and determined, and you will find your way.

HONOR YOUR SPIRIT

Imagine your spirit as a tiny caterpillar deep within you. Conscious breathing and a peaceful mind make up the cocoon your spirit needs to develop. Care for and nurture your spirit, and that tiny caterpillar will grow into a beautiful butterfly with a magnificent set of wings to carry you wherever you need to go. Do not be afraid of finding your true self.

LOVE YOURSELF

You are the only one who is with you from the moment you are born to the day you die. Cherish what you have. Realize your perfection. Understanding means grasping with the intellect, but realization is "knowing" within the body, mind, and spirit.

Seven Practical Truths for Becoming a Good Zen Yoga Adept

The amount of time you spend practicing Zen Yoga, or any other art for that matter, is not important. No one else in the world needs to be concerned about how much you give to it. Progress can come at any pace. Go at your own speed. Do what you can at the pace your body and mind allow. As you progress, your body will begin to feel and your mind will begin to know the benefits. Let this happen naturally.

Keep in mind these practical truths as you go.

1. Be Patient.
    It's a long journey. Rushing just gets you to the end faster. Then what?

2. Persevere.
    Continue training. Give yourself permission to feel better and better.

3. Do what you're able.
    It's not about what you can't do.

4. Find a Good Teacher.
    But learn from everyone.

5. Be a Good Teacher.
    Help others remember what they already know.

6. Meditate!
    Don't procrastinate!

7. Love it.
    Laugh and dance into eternity.

    ...and, of course, remember to breathe!

Continuing Zen Yoga Practice

Throughout your life advance daily,
becoming more skillful than yesterday,
more skillful than today. This is never ending.

—Yamamoto Tsunetomo

Zen Yoga Training Sheet

I have often found it useful to track my training progress over a period of time. Doing so has a number of benefits. First, it gives you a tangible record of the time and effort you are putting into your training. This can be invaluable as you work to build positive training habits; you can look back in a few months and see how you have progressed. You can decide where you have been consistent and where you may need to focus more attention. In addition, filling in check marks on the training sheet reinforces a sense of tangible accomplishment and enables you to establish and meet challenges to yourself.

Generating motivation is hard for many of us. The training sheet represents a commitment to practicing Zen Yoga and, therefore, is an implicit motivating factor that helps keep you focused as you track your progress. If you are genuinely committed to bettering yourself, the training sheet can be a valuable tool in assisting you to reach your goal.

The basic training sheet lists all of the primary Zen Yoga exercises. Simply place a check mark in the corresponding box on a day that you practice the exercise listed. Once you are accustomed to using it, you will want to adapt it to your own personal training habits. To this end, I have also included a blank training sheet that you can copy and modify to suit your needs.

Don't let this sheet intimidate you. If it helps in your Zen Yoga training, that is great. If it becomes a hassle or a burden, don't use it. It is simply another available tool.

MONTH																															
EXERCISE \ DATE	1	2	3	4	5	6	7	8	9	10	11	12	13	14	15	16	17	18	19	20	21	22	23	24	25	26	27	28	29	30	31
Cleansing Breath																															
Complete-Cycle Breathing																															
Microcosmic Orbit																															
Qigong																															
Bouncing																															
Circling																															
Lying-Down Stretching																															
Sitting Stretching																															
Kneeling Stretching																															
Standing Stretching																															
Inversions																															
Balance																															
Tension Release																															
Shake																															
Breath Walking																															

ZEN YOGA TRAINING SHEET

MONTH																																
EXERCISE / DATE	1	2	3	4	5	6	7	8	9	10	11	12	13	14	15	16	17	18	19	20	21	22	23	24	25	26	27	28	29	30	31

The Zen Yoga Daily Warm-Up

The Zen Yoga daily warm-up is an easy method of integrating Zen Yoga into daily life. It is a series of Zen Yoga exercises put together in a format that is simple to do and takes only twenty minutes each day. All of the exercises are done from a standing position and nothing is too difficult. The exercises are intended to raise your energy levels, loosen your joints, and assist in relaxing and easing tense or tight muscles.

The daily warm-up starts with breathing exercises. It is usually a good idea to start with these exercises in order to fill your body with the oxygen and energy you will use for the subsequent exercises. Start with a couple of Cleansing Breaths and practice some Opening Qigong and Gathering Qigong.

When you are ready, start at the hips, and begin rotating and circling your hip joints. It is always important to begin with the central torso. By waking up that part of the body you energize your core, and from there the energy spreads outward. Working on the torso, bend forward, back, and to the side. This is followed by Zen Squats.

Once your central core is warmed up, begin the Swan Qigong breathing exercise in order to center yourself and fill your body with more energy. The extremities are next: rotate your shoulders, arms, elbows, and wrists. Then move to the lower body and rotate your hips, knees, and ankles.

Once your body is loosened up, practice the Shake exercise. This will release any leftover tension. When you have finished the Shake exercise, practice the Energy Ball Qigong breathing exercise until you feel the energy moving smoothly through you.

Finally, once your body is warmed up, spend a short time working on the balance exercises.

The Zen Yoga daily warm-up is a quick and easy way to get yourself jump-started in the morning, and is also a good transition after a hard day of work. It recharges your body and clears your mind in a very short time. It is a quick and easy alternative to going to the gym, and takes much less time and effort.

The Zen Yoga daily warm-up is available on DVD at the Zen Yoga website at www.artofzenyoga.com

Conclusion

I hope that some part of this book has been helpful to you. I have no desire to make claims to any unique wisdom or knowledge. Many others before me have discovered the ideas I believe in and the techniques of practice. I simply wish to present them in a cohesive manner, in a language that is simple and clear.

I do believe that many of the problems we face could be alleviated by learning to breathe more effectively. It is ironic that the very tool we depend on to stay alive is also the key to a better existence on all levels, giving us mental clarity, peace, energy, hope, freedom, and vision. There are no tricks, no secrets; it is right there in front of us. And yet most of us will search for the answer everywhere else...gimmicks, diets, plans, pills...the more complicated the better. Why? Could it be that we consider ourselves different or better than nature itself; that to live in simple harmony, using what has been given us, is beneath us? Those are complex questions best left for another book. For now, let us be content with breathing, moving, stretching, and relaxing and see what changes occur.

To repeat it one last time, Zen is the condition of existing wholly in the immediate moment, inviting a new sense of self and holistic consciousness. It eliminates barriers and allows the individual to absorb the meaning of yoga immediately and with full understanding. Zen Yoga allows us to experience a sense of self that is open to the internal dynamics of personality as it functions in the present. The result is a mindfulness that draws on that sense of the moment and sets the stage for experiencing ourselves at the deepest spiritual level.

We are all on our own journey. But we are all connected by the universal energy that flows through us. If we are able to become more aware of that energy, maybe it will be possible for all of us to experience our spiritual nature not just individually, but as part of the unique collective known as the human race. For now, as you move along your path, I offer you blessings.

Peace.

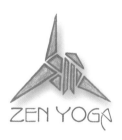

ZEN YOGA

APPENDIX 1

LIST OF EXERCISES

APPENDIX 2

LEVELS OF ZEN YOGA

Zen Yoga has been developed on a ranking system similar to some of the more traditional martial arts. Progression through different levels reflects the time and effort put into the training. How far one wishes to advance in rank is completely up to the individual. Age and physical ability are irrelevant as long as you are committed to your own personal growth. There is a place for everyone in Zen Yoga.

Each level has its own requirements. Certification of rank is provided after completion of the requirements for each level.

Zen Yoga Ranking System

■ **STUDENT**

Beginner Study Level

All participants in any Zen Yoga class are considered Zen Yoga students.

■ **ADEPT**

Intermediate Study Level

Zen Yoga adepts understand the basics of Zen Yoga and have begun to integrate them into their lives. Requirements: Completion of the Zen Yoga Fundamentals Course and the submission of a self-mastery project.

■ **INSTRUCTOR LEVEL 1**

Advanced study level

Level 1 Zen Yoga instructors are ready to begin teaching the basics of Zen Yoga to small groups and classes. Requirements: completion of adept-level program; one-on-one personal Zen Yoga training with sage-level instructor; completion of the Zen Yoga Instructor Training Course; organizing and hosting of a Zen Yoga workshop; and being able to teach the Zen Yoga daily warm-up effectively.

■ **INSTRUCTOR LEVEL 2**

Advanced study level

Level 2 Zen Yoga instructors are qualified to teach classes, workshops, and educational and corporate training programs. Requirements: completion of Instructor Level 1; teaching an organized Zen Yoga class (approximately one year); expanding their Zen Yoga community; organizing and hosting of a Zen Yoga workshop; completion of the Advanced Zen Yoga Course, including the submission of a personal holistic philosophy project.

■ SAGE LEVEL 1
Basic master level

Level 1 sages are in the process of expanding their knowledge base and adding to their own abilities. Requirements: completion of Instructor Level 2; teaching formal Zen Yoga class (approximately three years); training in hard- and soft-style martial arts; massage; yoga; or an equivalent art; organizing and hosting a Zen Yoga retreat; completion of the Zen Yoga Sage Course.

■ SAGE LEVEL 2
Intermediate master level

Level 2 sages have reached a high level of self-training and are able to create new Zen Yoga training methods. Requirements: completion of Sage Level 1; teaching Zen Yoga (including to children and seniors for five years); writing and publishing books and/or articles; creating innovative Zen Yoga training exercises; completion of the Zen Yoga Healer Course.

■ SAGE LEVEL 3
Advanced master level

Level 3 sages are highly skilled Zen Yoga teachers with a wide knowledge of many training methods. Requirements: completion of Sage Level 2; teaching Zen Yoga (approximately seven years); teaching Zen Yoga Instructor Course; and developing a Zen Yoga curriculum.

■ ZIN
Highest level of Zen Yoga mastery

ACKNOWLEDGMENTS

First of all I would like to thank Mom and Dad for just about everything. None of this would have been possible without them, their knowledge, and, of course, their wonderful editorial skills.

Thanks also to my instructors: Takayuki Mikami, Chien "King" Lam, Masatoshi Nakayama, and Shanti Gowans. And thanks to my many training partners: Rene Vildosola, Paul Carney, Damon Russell, Michel Berger, Jon Keeling and the Hoitsugan instructors, as well as all of the other people I have had the honor to be able to train with and learn from throughout this continuing journey.

I also must thank Joe Schoenig for first saying, "You should write this stuff down," all those years ago. And thanks to Aya Itagaki.

I especially want to thank my students and all those who have attended my various Zen Yoga workshops and events. You have made this book possible and I dedicate it to you.

In addition, I would like to thank Kevin, Sonia, Donna, Ellen, Joey, Carla and the rest of the Zen Yoga instructors and Adepts who have helped Zen Yoga to grow and expand. Also thanks to everyone at The Vershire Riding School, Beyond Care, and the Revive Wellness Center.

Thanks to my editor Barry Lancet and the group at Kodansha for getting behind this project and working to create a very special book.

And finally, a very special thanks to Rita for everything else, especially her willingness to become an integral part of this book and Zen Yoga as a whole.

（英文版）禅ヨガ

Zen Yoga: A Path to Enlightenment through Breathing, Movement and Meditation

2007 年 6 月 27 日　第 1 刷発行

著　者　アーロン・フーブス
発行者　富田　充
発行所　講談社インターナショナル株式会社
　　　　〒 112-8652 東京都文京区音羽 1-17-14
　　　　電話　03-3944-6493（編集部）
　　　　　　　03-3944-6492（マーケティング部・業務部）
　　　　ホームページ　www.kodansha-intl.com

印刷・製本所　大日本印刷株式会社

落丁本・乱丁本は購入書店名を明記のうえ、講談社インターナショナル業務部宛にお送りください。送料小社負担にてお取替えします。なお、この本についてのお問い合わせは、編集部宛にお願いいたします。本書の無断複写（コピー）、転載は著作権法の例外を除き、禁じられています。

定価はカバーに表示してあります。

© アーロン・フーブス 2007
Printed in Japan
ISBN 978-4-7700-3047-4